# OB/GYN Notes

First Edition

D1546205

**Roman T. Pachulski, MD**
Department of Medicine
Ottawa Civic Hospital
University of Ottawa
Ottawa, Canada

**APPLETON & LANGE**
Norwalk, Connecticut/San Mateo, California

Notice: Our knowledge in clinical sciences is constantly changing. As new information becomes available, changes in treatment and in the use of drugs become necessary. The author and the publisher of this volume have taken care to make certain that the doses of drugs and schedules of treatment are correct and compatible with the standards generally accepted at the time of publication. The reader is advised to consult carefully the instruction and information material included in the package insert of each drug or therapeutic agent before administration. This advice is especially important when using new or infrequently used drugs.

Copyright © 1990 by Appleton & Lange
A Publishing Division of Prentice Hall

90 91 92 93 94 / 10 9 8 7 6 5 4 3 2 1


Prentice Hall International (UK) Limited, *London*
Prentice Hall of Australia Pty. Limited, *Sydney*
Prentice Hall of Canada, Inc., *Toronto*
Prentice Hall Hispanoamericana, S.A., *Mexico*
Prentice Hall of India Private Limited, *New Delhi*
Prentice Hall of Japan, Inc., *Tokyo*
Simon & Schuster Asia Pte. Ltd., *Singapore*
Editora Prentice Hall do Brasil Ltda., *Rio de Janeiro*
Prentice Hall, *Englewood Cliffs, New Jersey*

**Library of Congress Cataloging-in-Publication Data**

Pachulski, R. (Roman), 1959–
    Ob/Gyn notes / R. Pachulski.
      p.  cm.
    ISBN 0-8385-6245-0
    1. Gynecology—Handbooks, manual, etc.  2. Obstetrics—Handbooks, manuals, etc.  [1. Family Planning—handbooks.  2. Genital Diseases, Female—handbooks.  3. Gynecology—handbooks.  4. Obstetrics—handbooks.  5. Pregnancy Complications—handbooks.]
    I. Title.  II. Title: Obstetrics/gynecology notes.
    [DNLM: WQ 39 P116o]
    RG110.P33  1990
    618—dc20                                                    89-17546
    DNLM/DLC                                                       CIP
    for Library of Congress


ISBN 0-8385-6245-0

PRINTED IN THE UNITED STATES OF AMERICA

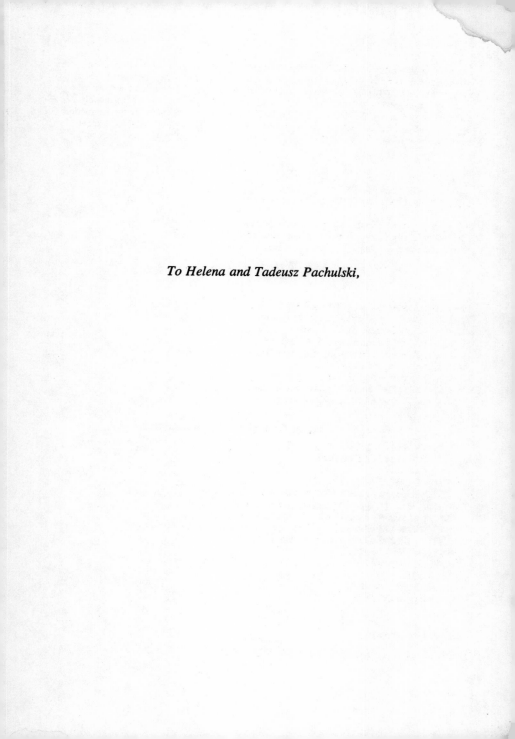

*To Helena and Tadeusz Pachulski,*

On that best portion of
      a good man's life,
His little, nameless,
      unremembered acts,
Of kindness and of love

W. Wordsworth

# Contents

Preface....................................................................ix
Acknowledgments......................................................xi

**CHAPTER 1 - BASIC SCIENCE**

GU Embryology................................................... 1

**CHAPTER 2 - NORMAL OBSTETRICS**

Physiological Changes in Pregnancy............................... 13
Hormones in Pregnancy.......................................... 16
Diagnosis of Pregnancy.......................................... 19
Prenatal Care................................................... 25
Labor.......................................................... 30
Neonatal Assessment............................................ 35
Puerperium..................................................... 38

**CHAPTER 3 - ABNORMAL OBSTETRICS**

Vaginal Bleeding and Pregnancy.................................. 43
Pregnancy-Induced Hypertension.................................. 53
Hemolytic Disease of the Newborn................................ 60
Medical Conditions in Pregnancy................................. 65
Evaluation of Fetal Well-Being.................................. 75
Ultrasound..................................................... 82
Dystocia....................................................... 84
Prolapse of the Umbilical Cord.................................. 89
Preterm Labor.................................................. 90
Multiple Pregnancy............................................. 97
Gestational Trophoblastic Disease.............................. 100
Obstetric Mortality........................................... 105

## CHAPTER 4 - GENERAL GYNECOLOGY

Vulvar Diseases........................................... 107
Vaginal Diseases.......................................... 117
Pelvic Pain (Secondary Dysmenorrhea)...................... 123
Uterovaginal Prolapse..................................... 137
Breast Carcinoma Screening................................ 139
Carcinoma of the Cervix................................... 141
Colposcopy................................................ 147
Leiomyoma................................................. 149
Endometrial Hyperplasia and Polyps........................ 153
Endometrial Carcinoma..................................... 157
Ovarian Neoplasia......................................... 160
Metastatic Tumors to the Ovary............................ 177

## CHAPTER 5 - REPRODUCTIVE GYNECOLOGY

Puberty................................................... 179
Menopause................................................. 181
Amenorrhea................................................ 184
Fertility................................................. 191
Dysfunctional Uterine Bleeding............................ 194
Dysmenorrhea.............................................. 202
Premenstrual Tension Syndrome............................. 203

## CHAPTER 6 - BIRTH CONTROL

Oral Contraceptive Pill................................... 205
Intrauterine Device....................................... 213
Summary of Reversible Contraceptive Methods............... 215
Sterilization............................................. 215
Induced Abortion.......................................... 218

## CHAPTER 7 - HUMAN SEXUALITY ........................... 223

## BIBLIOGRAPHY ........................................... 227

## INDEX ................................................. 229

# Preface

The intent of this book was to produce a handbook size volume that contains not only knee-jerk responses to specific questions but also an explanation for those responses. With the ever-increasing demand on a medical student's time such books must be brief. Voluminous books are all too often relegated to the bookshelf for lack of day-to-day pertinence. The basic premise for this series of texts is that large amounts of medical information are best assimilated when the underlying pathophysiology of the disorders is understood rather than memorizing many seemingly disparate facts.

# Acknowledgments

Many people provided counsel, support and encouragement during the writing of this manuscript. I wish to express my thanks to Dr. S. Jindal and Dr. R. Saginur for their encouragement at the outset of this endeavor. Dr. I. Hart and Dr. J. Bormanis helped secure for me some undisturbed time during which I could apply myself fully to the task at hand. I would also like to thank Dr. M. Bertrand for reviewing the section on gynecologic oncology. I would like to extend a special thanks to Dr. H. Muggah who, having reviewed the manuscript, provided insightful and constructive suggestions that have enriched these notes immeasurably. My thanks to R. Craig Percy and Chris Langan both of Appleton & Lange for their help and patience throughout this endeavor. George Pachulski was instrumental in helping me understand the world of microcomputers without which this endeavor would have been impossible. As always my love to Larysa Catherine.

# Basic Science

## GENITOURINARY EMBRYOLOGY

The development of the genital and urinary systems are intimately related. Congenital anomalies in one system are commonly associated with congenital anomalies in the other. Genitourinary embryology can be subdivided into five developmental units: (1) nephric unit (kidneys and ureters), (2) vesicourethral unit, (3) gonadal unit, (4) gonadal duct unit, and (5) external genitalia.

### Nephric Unit (See Fig. 1-1)

The nephric unit eventually consists of the ureters and the kidneys. The kidney develops as three successive pairs of excretory organs. The first primordial kidney is the nonfunctional **pronephros,** which appears early in the fourth week of gestation. The most lasting contribution of the pronephros is its drainage duct, the pronephric duct that later becomes the mesonephric duct. The second embryonic kidney or **mesonephros** is drained by the mesonephric (Wolffian) duct to the cloaca. The mesonephros is probably only transiently functional as an excretory organ in fetal life and degenerates by the eighth week of gestation. The mesonephric (Wolffian) duct develops into the gonadal duct system in men, but remains a vestigial structure in women. The **metanephros** or final functional kidney develops from the ureteric bud and metanephric mesenchyme. The ureteric bud (metanephric diverticulum), forms as an outgrowth from the caudal portion of the mesonephric duct (6 weeks' gestation) and forms the ureters, pelvis,

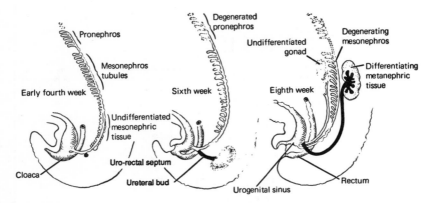

**Figure 1-1.** Schematic representation of the development of the nephric system. Only a few of the tubules of the pronephros are seen early in the fourth week, while the mesonephric tissue differentiates into mesonephric tubules that progressively join the mesonephric duct. The first sign of the ureteral bud from the mesonephric duct is seen. At 6 weeks, the pronephros has completely degenerated and the mesonephric tubules start to do so. The ureteral bud grows dorsocranially and has met the metanephric mesenchyme. At the eighth week, there is cranial migration of the differentiating metanephros. The cranial end of the ureteric bud expands and starts to show multiple successive outgrowths.
Adapted from *General Urology*, D.R. Smith, Lange Medical Publications.

calyces, and collecting tubules, while the metanephric mesenchyme forms the nephron (Bowman's capsule to distal convoluted tubule). The two units fuse to form a continuous uriniferous tubule that produces a functional excretory organ. The embryonic kidneys commence as pelvic organs whose hila are directed ventrally. They must ascend and rotate internally 90 degrees about their vertical axes to reach their final position.

Renal ectopy (e.g., pelvic kidney) or malrotation may occur if either ascent or internal rotation, respectively, are inadequate. Congenital ureteric malformations (e.g., ureteric duplication; bifid ureter) may result from imperfections of the metanephric diverticulum (ureteric bud). Neonatal polycystic kidney disease results when the collecting tubules (metanephric diverticulum) fail to become confluent with the nephrons (metanephric mesenchyme).

TABLE 1-1. UROGENITAL SINUS DEVELOPMENT

| Urogenital Sinus | Women | Men |
| --- | --- | --- |
| Vesicourethral canal | Bladder and entire urethra | Bladder and urethra superior to Wolffian insertion |
| Pelvic portion | | Remaining prostatic and membranous urethra |
| Phallic portion | Vagina | Proximal penile urethra (except glans) |

## Vesicourethral Unit

The urorectal septum divides the cloaca into a dorsal rectum and a ventral urogenital sinus. The urogenital sinus is divided into three components: (1) the cranial vesicourethral canal, (2) the middle pelvic portion, and (3) the caudal phallic portion. The urogenital sinus develops as described in Table 1-1.

The hymen is a vestigial membrane that separates the vaginal lumen from the introital vestibule. The wolffian ducts and the ureters gain separate access to the vesicourethral canal as the caudal wolffian duct is absorbed into the trigone. The allantois becomes a thick tube (urachus) that subsequently involutes to form the medial umbilical ligament. The prostate develops from urethral epithelial cord outgrowths above and below the orifices of the wolffian ducts.

Failure of the urorectal septum to divide the cloaca appropriately may result in a persistent cloaca, a rectovesical fistula, or a rectourethral fistula. Anomalous or incomplete urachal degeneration may lead to the formation of a small urachal diverticulum or a frank vesicoumbilical fistula. If the genital primordia arise caudad to the orifice of the urogenital sinus, epispadias with exstrophy of the bladder may occur.

## Gonadal Unit

Chromosomal sex (either 46-X,Y or 46-X,X) determines gonadal sex, which subsequently governs somatic sex (gonadal ducts and external genitalia).

**TABLE 1–2. SUMMARY OF GONADAL DEVELOPMENT**

| Site of Origin | Primordial Tissue | Mature Derivatives[a] |
|---|---|---|
| Mesonephros | Gonadal mesenchyme | Theca interna/Leydig's cells |
| Yolk sac endoderm | Primordial germ cells | Oogonia/spermatogonia |
| Gonadal ridge | Coelomic epithelium | Granulosa/Sertoli |

[a]Female/male.

Gonads develop from three components: (1) the specialized gonadal mesenchyme of the mesonephros, (2) the coelomic epithelium, and (3) yolk sac endoderm (Table 1-2). The specialized gonadal mesenchyme of the mesonephros forms the gonadal stroma, which in men includes Leydig's cells (site of gonadal testosterone synthesis) and in women includes theca interna cells. The yolk sac endoderm is the site of initial formation (fourth week of gestation) of the primordial germ cells that are subsequently incorporated into coelomic epithelial structures where the germs cells develop into spermatogonia (men) or oogonia (women). The coelomic epithelium proliferates to form the gonadal ridge ventromedial to the nephrogenic cords and gives rise to the primary and secondary sex cords. (Fig. 1-2) These primary sex cords degenerate in women, while in men they incorporate the primordial germ cells and form the seminiferous tubules. The Sertoli support cells of the seminiferous tubules are the coelomic epithelial derivatives in the mature male gonad (testis). The secondary sex cords only form in the female fetus. The secondary sex cords incorporate the primordial germ cells and form primordial follicles. The granulosa cells (site of gonadal estradiol synthesis) are the coelomic epithelial derivatives in the mature female gonad (ovary). (Fig. 1-3)

The primary sex cords are also called medullary sex cords because they lose contact with the gonadal cortical surface and drain toward the medullary Wolffian duct. The secondary sex cords are also called the cortical sex cords because they retain contact with the gonadal cortex where the follicles empty during ovulation. The **indifferent gonad** refers to the multipotential primordial gonad identifiable between the sixth and eighth weeks of gestation. Definitive identification of a male gonad is first possible at ~7 weeks' gestation when the tunica albuginea forms at the gonadal cortex.

The primordial gonad forms retroperitoneally in the dorsal wall of the

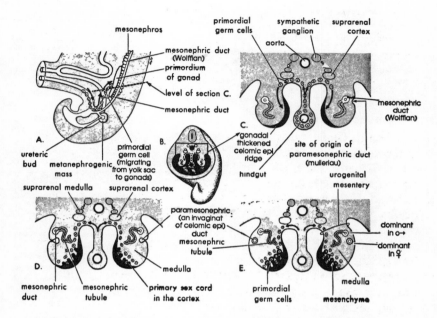

**Figure 1-2.** A, Sketch of five-week embryo illustrating the migration of primordial germ cells. B, Three-dimensional sketch of the caudal region of a five-week embryo showing the location and extent of the gonadal ridges on the medial aspect of the urogenital ridges. C, Transverse section showing the primordium of the adrenal glands, the gonadal ridges, and the migration of primordial germ cells.

Adapted from *The Developing Human 2/E*, K.L. Moore, W.B. Saunders Company.

main peritoneal cavity. Mature gonads are located more caudally within the pelvis (ovary) or in the scrotum (male). The caudad gonadal migration follows the path of the retroperitoneal fibromuscular gubernaculum. The gubernaculum extends from the inferior pole of the gonad into the processus vaginalis of the labioscrotal swelling. In men the gonad descends (~7 months' gestational age) the complete length of the gubernaculum into the scrotum. The gubernaculum then degenerates. Free communication between the main peritoneal cavity and the scrotum is obliterated as the processus

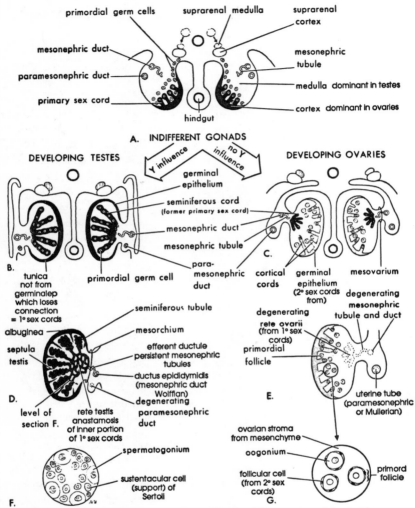

**Figure 1-3.** Schematic sections illustrating the differentiation of the indifferent gonads into testes or ovaries. *A*, Six weeks, showing the indifferent gonads composed of an outer cortex and an inner medulla. *B*, Seven weeks, showing testes developing under the influence of a Y chromosome. Note that the primary sex cords have become seminiferous cords and that they are separated from the surface epithelium by the tunica albuginea. *C*, 12 weeks, showing ovaries beginning to develop in the absence of a Y chromo-

vaginalis involutes. In women the gonad descends only partially down the gubernaculum whose remnants persist as the ovarian ligament (between the ovary and the uterus) and the round ligament (between the uterus and the labia majora).

Gonadal agenesis or hypogenesis results when the gonadal development fails. Cryptorchidism refers to arrested gonadal descent along the normal path of the gubernaculum; gonadal ectopy refers to gonadal position other than expected at maturity or during normal descent. Incomplete obliteration of the processus vaginalis can result in hydrocele (male) formation or development of Nuck's canal cyst (female).

## Gonadal Duct Unit

In men the Wolffian (mesonephric) duct predominates and gives rise to the vas deferens, seminal vesicles, and ejaculatory ducts. The mesonephric tubules fuse to give the efferent ductules and the epididymis. In women the müllerian (paramesonephric) duct system predominates forming the fallopian tubes, the corpus, and the cervix uteri. The müllerian ducts originate as invaginations of the coelomic epithelium on the lateral surface of the urogenital ridge (see Fig. 1-3). Functional testicular tissue produces testosterone and müllerian inhibiting factor (MIF) that promotes ipsilateral male development of the gonadal ducts. Absent or dysfunctional testes result in ipsilateral female gonadal duct development. Testosterone promotes ipsilateral persistence of the wolffian ducts; MIF causes degeneration of the ipsilateral müllerian ducts.

---

some influence. Cortical cords have extended from the surface epithelium, displacing the primary sex cords centrally into the mesovarium, where they form the rudimentary rete ovarii. *D,* Testis at 20 weeks, showing the rate testis and the seminiferous tubules derived from the seminiferous cords. An efferent ductule has developed from a mesonephric tubule, and the mesonephric duct has become the duct of the epididymis. *E,* Ovary at 20 weeks, showing the primordial follicles formed from the cortical cords. The rete ovarii derived from the primary sex cords and the mesonephric tubule and duct are regressing. *F,* Section of a seminiferous tubule from a 20-week fetus. Note that no lumen is present at this stage, and that the seminiferous epithelium is composed of two kinds of cells. *G,* Section from the ovarian cortex of a 20-week fetus showing three primordial follicles.
Adapted from *The Developing Human 2/E,* K.L. Moore, W.B. Saunders Company.

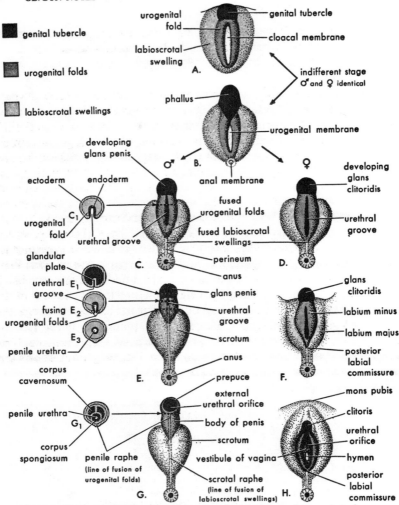

**Figure 1-4.** *A* and *B,* Diagrams illustrating development of the external genitalia during the indifferent stage (four to seven weeks). *C, E,* and *G,* Stages in the development of male external genitalia at about 9, 11, and 12 weeks, respectively. To the left are schematic transverse sections (*C₁, E₁* to *E₃,* and *G₁*) through the developing penis illustrating formation of the spongy urethra. *D, F,* and *H,* Stages in the development of female external genitalia at 9, 11, and 12 weeks, respectively.

Adapted from *The Developing Human 2/E,* K.L. Moore, W.B. Saunders Company.

Numerous anatomic variations of the uterus (e.g., bifid, reduplication) are possible as the result of incomplete midline müllerian duct fusion.

## External Genitalia

The labioscrotal swellings, urogenital folds, and genital tubercle develop into female external genitalia in the absence of an ipsilateral testis. Prenatal virilization of a male fetus is accomplished by dihydrotestosterone (DHT) (Fig. 1-4). The primordial end-organs (labioscrotal swellings, urogenital folds, genital tubercle) possess testosterone receptors with 5-alpha reductase activity capable of catalyzing testosterone conversion to the active virilizing agent DHT. Pubertal virilization is accomplished through the direct action of testosterone on the immature genitalia. The pubertal rise in testosterone levels is stimulated by a surge in luteinizing hormone (LH) levels.

Maldevelopment of the gonads, gonadal ducts, and external genitalia may result in *pseudohermaphroditism*. Pseudohermaphroditism is defined as somatic sex inappropriate (in whole or in part) for gonadal sex. *True hermaphroditism* is the presence of the gonads of both sexes in one individual and is extremely rare. Any inconsistencies between the presumed sex of an infant and the appearance of external genitalia should prompt investigation for pseudohermaphroditism. Early diagnosis may obviate gender identity problems for the child by permitting early therapeutic interventions. The Klebs classification for pseudohermaphroditism defines gonadal sex on the basis of microscopic examination of the gonad (Table 1-3).

**TABLE 1-3. ABBREVIATED CLASSIFICATION OF FEMALE PSEUDOHERMAPHRODITISM**

1. *Virilizing Adrenal Enzyme Deficiencies*
   21-hydroxylase[a]   9 5 %
   ⎰11-beta hydroxylase[b]
   ⎱17-alpha hydroxylase[b]
   3-beta hydroxysteroid dehydrogenase[a]

2. *Prenatal Exposure to Maternal Androgens*
   Androgenic ovarian tumors (rare)
   Luteoma of pregnancy
   Androgenic adrenal tumour

[a]Salt wasting; [b]salt retaining.

The most common causes of female pseudohermaphroditism are the virilizing adrenal enzyme deficiencies. Ninety-five percent of these cases are due to 21-hydroxylase deficiency (autosomal recessive). Adrenal enzyme deficiencies, which block cortisol synthesis as well as sex steroid production (Fig. 1-5), abrogate cortisol-mediated negative feedback on the hypothalamus and pituitary. The latter two glands then produce unrestrained amounts of corticotropin-releasing hormone (CRH) and adrenocorticotropic

95%

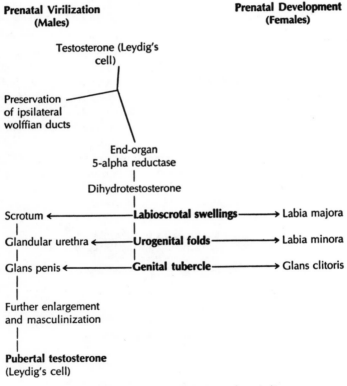

Figure 1-5. Somatic sex—external genitalia.

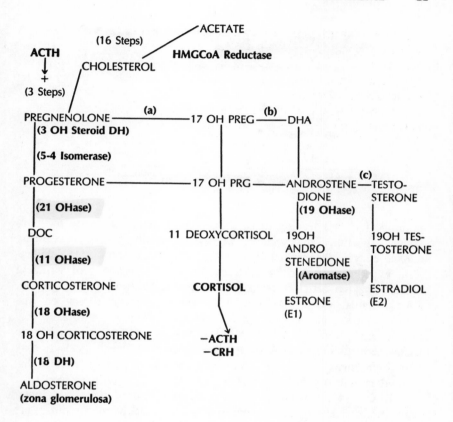

(a) 17 OHase (not found in zona glomerulosa); (b) 17-20 Desmolase; (c) 17 Ketosteroid Reductase.
**ACTH,** adrenocorticotropic hormone; **CRH,** corticotropin releasing hormone; **DH,** dehydrogenase; **DHA,** dehydroepiandrosterone; **DOC,** deoxycorticosterone; **OH,** hydroxy(1); **PREG,** pregnenolone; **PROG,** progesterone

**Figure 1-6.** Adrenal steroid synthesis.

**TABLE 1-4. ABBREVIATED CLASSIFICATION OF MALE PSEUDOHERMAPHRODITISM**

1. *Hypotestosteronemic Gonadal Enzyme Deficiencies*
   3-beta hydroxysteroid dehydrogenase
   17-alpha hydroxylase
   17,20-desmolase
   17-ketosteroid reductase
2. *End-Organ Defects*
   Androgen insensitivity syndrome[a]
   5-alpha reductase deficiency[b]

[a]Formerly testicular feminization syndrome.
[b]Variable masculinization at puberty.

hormone (ACTH) leading to adrenocortical hyperplasia (hence the term congenital adrenal hyperplasia). Severe salt-wasting forms of virilizing adrenal enzyme deficiencies may present shortly after birth with dehydration, hyperkalemia, and hyponatremia; salt-retaining forms of virilizing adrenal enzyme deficiencies may be suspected because of hypertension, hypernatremia, and hypokalemia. Treatment of virilizing adrenal enzyme deficiency involves supplementation with physiologic doses of glucocorticoid, e.g., cortisone, 37.5 mg/day PO or its equivalent. Female pseudohermaphroditism due to prenatal maternal androgen exposure may feminize normally at puberty with ovulatory menstrual periods provided that the müllerian duct system is intact.

Table 1-4 gives an abbreviated classification of male pseudohermaphroditism. The remaining causes of male pseudohermaphroditism are very rare. Male pseudohermaphroditism (with the exception of androgen insensitivity syndrome, X-linked recessive) usually results from autosomal recessive mutations. Note that gonadal testosterone synthesis is accomplished by the same pathways as adrenal steroid synthesis. Gonadal enzyme deficiency syndromes are not associated with salt or water aberrations or adrenal hyperplasia. Most (80%) male pseudohermaphrodites have genitalia more consistent with female anatomy, therefore, management consists of the removal of ectopic testes (prone to malignant degeneration), functional and cosmetic modification of the external genitalia, female sex steroid supplementation from puberty on, and periodic endometrial biopsy.

# 2

# Normal Obstetrics

## PHYSIOLOGIC CHANGES IN PREGNANCY

The physiologic alterations of pregnancy are not pathologic but they are nonetheless significant. The following discussion is divided according to the pertinent major organ systems.

### General Comments

During the course of normal pregnancy there is a 12±4-kg weight gain. Solid organs account for 6.75 kg, whereas the remainder is attributable to the increase in total body water (TBW) both extracellular (ECF) and intracellular (ICF) fluid

| | |
|---|---|
| Fetus | 3.5 kg |
| Placenta | 0.75 kg |
| Uterus | 1.0 kg |
| Breasts | 1.5 kg |
| ECF volume | 5.25 kg |

Not surprisingly the mother is in a general anabolic state characterized by: (1) a 15% increase in oxygen consumption, (2) a positive nitrogen balance, (3) an energy requirement increase to ~40 kcal/kg/day during pregnancy, ~45 kcal/kg/day during lactation, and (4) an increase in the basal metabolic rate (BMR) by 10% to 15%.

### Skin and Skin Appendages

See the section on diagnosis of pregnancy.

13

## Respiratory System

There is an increased sensitivity of the central nervous system (CNS) respiratory center to the partial arterial pressure of carbon dioxide (Pa $CO_2$) which may be due to increased progesterone levels. There is a 40% increase in the tidal volume and the minute volume. Progesterone, with its smooth muscle relaxant properties, may also be responsible for the ~35% increase in cross-sectional diameter of the airways. The expanding uterus results in upward displacement of the diaphragm and a decline in the functional residual capacity (FRC). This improves somewhat with lightening.

## Cardiovascular System

The factors that govern systemic blood pressure are briefly summarized in Figure 2-1. During pregnancy several of these factors are altered in ways that are antagonistic to one another.

Throughout the course of the pregnancy the progestational vascular smooth muscle spasmolytic effect is relatively constant. It is this mechanism that underlies a decreased venous return and, therefore, a decline in the end diastolic pressure (EDP), (i.e., increased venous pooling). It also causes a decrease in total peripheral resistance (TPR) by way of arterial vasodilatation. These changes act to decrease the blood pressure.

Estrogen, as outlined in the section on oral contraceptive pills acts to promote hypertension through increased reninangiotensin aldosterone (R/A/A) system mediated fluid/electrolyte retention (increased blood volume (BV) and EDP). The protein anabolic property of estrogen acts to increase the plasma protein content. This effect is, however, literally drowned out by fluid retention. The plasma protein concentration actually declines by ~15%.

The progestational effect on EDP antagonizes that of estrogen, the former decreases venous return, the latter increases blood volume. The net effect is an increase in preload. In addition, pregnancy is characterized by increased heart rate ~20%.

During the first and second trimesters the upper limit of normal for blood pressure (130/80) is lower than that of the general population indicating predominance of the progestational effects; in the third trimester, however, the upper limit of normal returns to that which is accepted for the

↑ Plasma Protein Content, but [PP] actually ↓

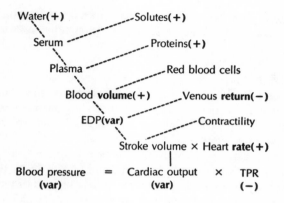

Water(+)                    Solutes(+)

Serum                       Proteins(+)

Plasma                      Red blood cells

Blood volume(+)         Venous return(−)

EDP(var)                     Contractility

Stroke volume × Heart rate(+)

Blood pressure    =    Cardiac output    ×    TPR
  (var)                    (var)                  (−)

+, increased; −, decreased; **EDP,** end diastolic pressure; **TPR,** total peripheral resistance; **Var,** Variable changes during pregnancy.

**Figure 2-1.** Determinants of systemic blood pressure.

general nonpregnant population (140/90). Thus during the third trimester the opposing influences balance one another.

## Gastrointestinal and Genitourinary Systems

Pica, cravings for unusual foodstuffs, is a greatly celebrated trait of pregnancy. Swollen or bleeding gums are also quite common and most often self-limited. Nausea, with or without emesis, is thought to be at least in part due to progestational relaxation of the smooth muscle of the lower esophageal sphincter (LES). A similar action on the large bowel results in constipation.

Fluid retention has already been discussed. The increase in blood volume increases both the renal blood flow (RBF) and the glomerular filtration rate (GFR). The inherent increase in filtered fraction (FF = GFR × Plasma concentration) of a solute (e.g., glucose) may overwhelm the renal threshold for resorption of various solutes. For this reason glycosuria is an unreliable test for diabetes mellitus in pregnancy.

Symptoms of bladder irritation (urgency, frequency) may also occur due to uterine compression. Stasis and reflux in the genitourinary tract is promoted by progestins. Dextrorotation of the uterus mechanically enhances this effect on the right ureter, thus preferentially promoting right-sided pyelonephritis.

## Musculoskeletal & Blood
Lumbar lordosis toward the latter half of term is a secondary postural change to compensate for the new center of gravity. The general ligamentous laxity seen during pregnancy is especially useful at the symphysis and the sacro-coccygeal regions during delivery.

The dilutional effect of excess body fluid lowers the hematocrit and hemoglobin concentration. The white blood cell count (7.5 to 15 × 1000) rises as does the platelet count. A generalized increase in the risk of thrombosis attributed to estrogen (see oral contraceptive pill section) in addition to the pelvic venous compression promotes lower limb thrombophlebitis (in both deep and superficial systems).

## Endocrine System
(See section on hormones in pregnancy.) There is an estrogen-mediated increase in both uterine size and oxytocin responsiveness. Elevations of cortisol and other anti-insulin hormones stresses the available insulin reserve, in some cases resulting in gestational diabetes. Parathormone (PTH) levels rise permitting relative maternal demineralization, increasing the $Ca^{++}$ available for the forming fetal skeleton.

## HORMONES IN PREGNANCY

### Pituitary Gland
Luteinizing hormone (LH) from the adenohypophysis supports the corpus luteum as usual during the latter half of the 28-day ovulatory cycle whether the egg is fertilized or not. This maintains the estrogen (EST) and especially progesterone (PROGEST) synthesis in the corpus luteum.

At about 8 weeks from the last menstrual period (LMP) the pituitary production of adrenocorticotropic hormone (ACTH) and melanocyte stim-

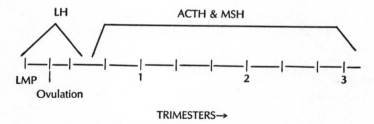

**Figure 2-2.** Pituitary hormone production in pregnancy.

ulating hormone (MSH) rises (Fig. 2-2). This coincides with the pigmentary changes associated with pregnancy as well as stria formation.

## Placenta

If pregnancy is achieved, the newly forming fetal organ, the placenta, takes over the gonadotropic function of the pituitary. The hormone responsible for this is human or placental chorionic gonadotropin (HCG or PCG). Placental HCG production declines after the first trimester and the corpus luteum involutes. The loss of the corpus luteum does not signify the loss of estrogen or progesterone synthesis, these are now made directly by the maturing placenta (Fig. 2-3).

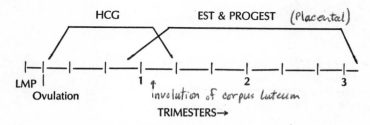

**Figure 2-3.** Placental hormone production in pregnancy.

hCG Functionally similar
to LH

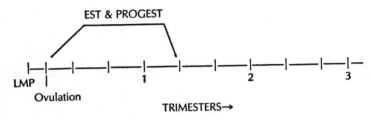

**EST & PROGEST**

LMP
Ovulation
1     2     3
TRIMESTERS→

**Figure 2-4.** Corpus luteum hormone production in pregnancy.

## Corpus Luteum

The corpus luteum is the source of the female sex steroids (estrogen and progesterone) during the latter half of each ovulatory cycle (supported by pituitary gonadotropins) and during the first trimester (supported by placental gonadotropins). HCG is functionally very similar to LH. By the end of the first trimester gonadotropin synthesis ceases and the corpus luteum involutes (Fig. 2-4).

## Adrenal Cortex

The adrenal cortex responds to the increased secretion of pituitary ACTH with an increase in glucocorticoid production. This accounts for several of the skin changes normally seen in pregnancy (e.g., stria formation) (Fig. 2-5).

Figure 2-6 is a more complete profile of placental hormone synthesis during pregnancy.

Adrenal Cortex

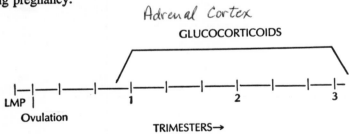

**GLUCOCORTICOIDS**

LMP
Ovulation
1     2     3
TRIMESTERS→

**Figure 2-5.** Glucocorticoid production in pregnancy.

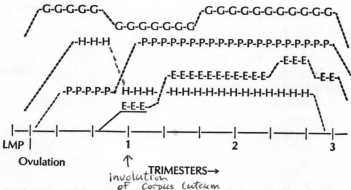

G, glucocorticoids; H, human chorionic gonadotropin; P, progesterone; E, Estrogen.

**Figure 2-6.** Placental hormone synthesis.

# DIAGNOSIS OF PREGNANCY

The diagnosis of pregnancy is classically based on signs and symptoms divided into groups labeled presumptive, probable, and positive evidence.

## Presumptive Evidence
Signs
    Secondary amenorrhea
    Breast changes
    Vaginal discoloration
    Skin pigmentation/striae  *msH*
Symptoms
    Sensation of pregnancy
    Nausea  *Prog mediated relaxation of LES of esoph.*
    Bladder irritability  *stasis of GU mediated by prog*
    Quickening  *16–20 wks*

As mentioned in the section discussing amenorrhea, any woman experiencing cessation of regular periods must be considered pregnant until proven otherwise.

Breast changes include: (1) dilatation of superficial veins; (2) areolar enlargement and hyperpigmentation; (3) enlargement of breast parenchyme; (4) increased prominence of the periareolar sebaceous glands, **Montgomery's tubercles** (may be present during the latter half of any menstrual cycle); (5) colostrum production; and (6) symptomatic changes (tingling, soreness, heaviness).

Vaginal mucosal discoloration, **Chadwick's sign,** is the result of vascular congestion. It manifests at the cervix and vulva as well. The violaceous hue appears at about the sixth to eighth week LMP but may occur with any condition causing pelvic vascular engorgement (e.g., pelvic mass lesion).

Changes in skin pigmentation and the formation of striae are manifestations of excess glucocorticoid, estrogen, progesterone, and melanin stimulating hormone (MSH). The bulk of the glucocorticoid is produced in the adrenal cortex in response to increase pituitary ACTH synthesis starting at about 8 weeks LMP.

Certain sites have a predeliction for hyperpigmentation: (1) **chloasma** (also known as melasma or "mask of pregnancy") facial hyperpigmentation, rare but relatively irreversible; (2) hyperpigmentation of the midline abdominal skin, **"linea nigra";** (3) areolar, perineal, and axilary areas; (4) any newly forming scars during pregnancy; and (5) preexisting nevi. Nevi may also arise de novo during pregnancy. Skin hyperpigmentation persists postpartum.

Superficial vascular changes are the result of unknown estrogenic effects as well as progestationally induced smooth muscle relaxation. **Spider angiomata, palmar erythema,** and rarely **granuloma gravidarum** (a hemangioma found in the oral cavity) are attributed to estrogen. A combination of the effect of progesterone and uterine vascular compression promote lower limb and perianal **venous varicosities.** Vascular changes of pregnancy are reversible.

**Atrophic striae** (purplish scarlike lesions that later become white) may occur on the thighs, abdomen, buttocks, and breasts due to the weakening of

*Quickening  16-20 wks*

underlying elastic tissues. **Striae gravidarum** (atrophic striae developing during pregnancy) may fade, but rarely disappear entirely.

Other possible skin and skin appendage changes include: (1) **molluscum fibrosum gravidarum,** benign skin papillomas on the neck and upper chest; (2) self-limited **gingivitis;** (3) increased perspiration due to the increase in estrogen responsive eccrine sweat glands; (4) **telogen effluvium** (a postpartum event), the loss of up to 30% of scalp hair in the first 3 months after delivery (usually replaced with new hair); and (5) increased likelihood of **vaginitides** (trichomonal, candidal) due to vaginal pH changes.

The subjective sensation of pregnancy is something that can be relied upon in the multiparous woman. Unfortunately the timing of this symptom is unpredictable, and therefore it rarely helps make the diagnosis of pregnancy.

**Nausea** with or without **emesis** is a relatively common occurrence in the first trimester. Due in part to the laxity of the LES promoted by progesterone. This entity tends to be worse early in the day (morning sickness). If very severe before 20 weeks LMP one should be suspicious of molar pregnancy; if it persists beyond that time, multiple pregnancy should be considered.

Symptoms of **urinary bladder irritatability** (frequency, urgency, dysuria) have a bimodal distribution: early in the first trimester due to direct uterine compression and in the third trimester when lightening occurs and the presenting fetal part descends.

**Quickening** refers to the mother's initial perception of fetal movement. This tends to occur around the 16th to 20th week LMP. Again multiparous women notice this earlier than primigravidas.

## Probable Evidence
Signs
Abdominal enlargement
Uterine changes
(size, Hegar, Piskacek)
Cervical changes
(Goodell, Chadwick)

> Hegar's sign = palpable softening of lower portion of t/ uterine corpus
>
> Piskacek's = unilat soft prominence at the cornu that occurs if nidation is assymetric

Ballottement
Outlining fetal parts
Symptoms
  Abdominal distension
  Braxton-Hicks contraction
Laboratory
  Endocrine tests
  Hemagglutination inhibition (HAI)
  Latex flocculation inhibition (LFI)
  Radioimmunoassay (RIA)
  Bioassay

Abdominal enlargement becomes clinically apparent at ~20 weeks LMP, whereas symptomatic abdominal distension occurs earlier.

As pregnancy progresses the uterus enlarges to accommodate its growing passenger. Before the uterus ascends beyond the pelvic inlet, the estimation of its size is quite subjective but after the 20th week LMP it is objectively quantified as the **symphisis–fundal height** (SFH) (Table 2-1).

Palpable alterations in uterine consistency and shape have been given eponyms: **Hegar's sign** is the palpable softening of the lower portion of the uterine corpus; **Piskacek's sign** refers to a detectable unilateral soft prominence at the cornu that occurs if nidation is asymmetric. Both signs occur at

TABLE 2-1. SYMPHISIS–FUNDAL HEIGHT AND GESTATIONAL AGE

| Gestational Age (wk LMP) | Pelvic Examination (<20 wk) | SFH(>20wk) |
|---|---|---|
| 6 | "Plum-size" | |
| 8 | "Peach-size" | |
| 12 | "Orange-size" | |
| 16 | "Grapefruit-size" | |
| 20 | | Uterine Fundus at umbilicus |
| 20–36 | | ↑ 1 cm/wk |
| 36–38 | | Xiphisternum |
| 38–40 | | 2 cm descent at lightening |

Goodell's sign = Δ in cervical consistency from firm to soft.

NORMAL OBSTETRICS    23

about **6 weeks LMP,** however, the latter is only useful if it was previously known that there were no subserosal myomas.

Cervical changes include Chadwick's sign and **Goodell's sign;** a change in cervical consistency from firm to soft.

Ballottement is performed abdominally or per vaginum at about mid-pregnancy when the fetus is relatively small compared with the contents of the amniotic sac and floats freely. The palpating fingers push abruptly against the adjacent fetal part causing that part to recede and quickly return. This is a nonspecific test that detects free-floating objects (e.g., mass lesion within ascitic fluid).

Palpation of distinct fetal parts becomes possible in the latter half of pregnancy as they abut the abdominal wall more closely. Occasionally subserous myomas have been mistaken for pregnancy.

Pregnancy tests, whether analyses of urine, blood, or bioassay are designed to detect HCG. They do **not** constitute positive evidence of pregnancy because most HCG assays are relatively nonspecific. Three pituitary glycohormones LH, FSH, and TSH possess alpha and beta subunits, as does HCG. The alpha subunits of all these hormones are structurally identical, therefore assays capable of recognizing alpha subunits cannot distinguish between these 4 hormones. The beta subunits of these hormones are structurally dissimilar, thus the beta-HCG RIA test, which employs only antibodies to the beta subunit, is specific for the placental HCG. HCG production begins very early, possibly even before nidation. This assay reaches levels consistent with the diagnosis of pregnancy 8 to 9 days after ovulation (provided conception has occurred) or about 21 days from LMP.

The quantitative nature of this assay lends itself particularly well to the evaluation of ectopic pregnancy as well as follow-up of gestational trophoblastic disease. This will be discussed in further detail in the appropriate sections.

Both LFI and HAI urine tests are based on the same premise; anti-HCG antibody is added to the sample urine followed by addition of HCG laden red blood cells (HAI) or latex particles (LFI) with subsequent observation to see if there is clumping or not (Table 2-2).

If HCG is present in the urine sample it removes the added anti-HCG antibody before the anti-HCG antibody can interact with the marker-

*Braxton- Hicks contractions =
occur anytime during pregnancy*

TABLE 2-2. URINE TESTS FOR PREGNANCY

| Urine Sample | Test Result | Interpretation |
|---|---|---|
| HCG present | No clumping | Pregnant |
| HCG absent | Clumping occurs | Not pregnant |

absorbed HCG (either red blood cells or latex particles laden with HCG). These tests are not reliable before 42 days LMP (28 days after conception).

**Braxton–Hicks** contractions are intermitent, irregular, painless uterine contractions that occur any time between nidation and onset of true labor. They can also be produced by other forms of uterine irritation, e.g., myoma, hematometra.

## Positive Evidence
Signs
Detection of distinct fetal heart rate by the examiner
Perception of fetal motion by the examiner
Symptoms
Laboratory
Ultrasound
Radiologic examination

A gestational sac can be detected as early as the fifth week LMP and fetal heart activity can be noted by real time ultrasound (U/S) studies as early as 7 weeks LMP; clinically it is not heard until the 10th to 12th week LMP by Doppler or ~18 weeks LMP by stethoscope. Some time after 20 weeks LMP fetal movements become palpable to the examiner.

Radiographic examination is rarely indicated at present and should be avoided in the first trimester. Radiographs may be useful (primarily during labor) to diagnose difficult presentations.

**Pseudocyesis** or imaginary pregnancy is occasionally seen in perimenopausal women with strong unfulfilled desires of motherhood. It is characterized by the presence of the appropriate symptoms but few if any signs of pregnancy.

The duration of pregnancy is usually estimated by the duration of time

*Nagele's rule :  LMP + 1 yr + 1 wk - 3 mos.*
*EDC*

*Spalding's Sign = overlapping cranial bones by X-ray*

elapsed since the first day of the last regular menstrual period, recorded as weeks LMP. Conception in fact cannot occur before ovulation, thus this method falsely extends the duration of pregnancy by roughly 2 weeks. Nevertheless it represents the accepted convention by which pregnancy is said to be 40 weeks LMP (265 days gestation plus 15 days) in duration. The probable date of delivery or in more archaic terms the **estimated date of confinement** (EDC) can be calculated by **Nagele's rule: LMP + 1 year + 1 week − 3 months.**

## Fetal Death

In addition to the ultrasound evidence listed elsewhere the following factors are suggestive of fetal morbidity or death: (1) absent or slower than expected increase in uterine size, (2) cessation of fetal movement, (3) laboratory pregnancy tests revert to negativity, (4) declining plasma estriol levels, and (5) declining insulin requirements in a mother with diabetes mellitus. **Spalding's sign,** overlapping cranial bones visualized on radiographic studies, is highly suggestive of fetal death. Disseminated intravascular coagulation may complicate fetal death especially if the fetus is not promptly expelled or removed from the uterus.

## PRENATAL CARE

A full history and Physical Examination is obtained on the initial visit. Specific areas of interest include menstrual and previous childbearing history. The establishment of the usual volume and duration of menses, as well as the interval separating them, permits the establishment of an expected date of delivery. The reliability of this estimate depends primarily on regularity of prior menstrual periods.

Prior pregnancies and their outcomes can be concisely recorded in the following fashion. One lists five pertinent bits of information in a conventional manner:

- **G—Gravidity:** The total number of pregnancies regardless of their duration or number of infants per pregnancy. This will be the sum of the next three categories T, P, and A.

- *T—Term Births:* These are defined as pregnancies carried for longer than 37 but less than 42 weeks since LMP.
- *P—Preterm Births:* These are defined as pregnancies carried for longer than 20 but less than 37 weeks since LMP.
- *A—Aborted Pregnancies:* Any pregnancy terminated before 20 weeks LMP whether spontaneous or induced.
- *L—Live Births:* Any infant that shows evidence of spontaneous respiration, cardiac activity, movement of voluntary muscles, or other signs of life after birth (see obstetric mortality section).

Historical data concerning chronic medical illness should also be recorded. Routine evaluation of vital signs and weight are critical for the early detection of pregnancy-induced hypertension (PIH) and inadequate weight gain suggestive of intrauterine growth retardation (IUGR). **Excessive weight gain** may suggest PIH, fetal macrosomia, or polyhydramnios. Evaluation of the **SFH** by the physician and fetal movement by the mother are helpful clinical adjuncts in determining fetal well-being.

The initial laboratory investigations consist primarily of pertinent screening studies. **(1) Blood tests:** (a) hemoglobin hematocrit (Hb/Hct) to detect anemia. The dilutional nadir in the Hb level occurs between the 28th to 32nd week LMP; a value less than 110 g/L is significant. These studies are performed at the initial visit, at about the 30th week LMP, and then finally near term. (b) A/B/O and Rh blood group typing is indicated for both parents. (c) A screen for atypical red blood cell surface antigens (performed as part of the routine blood typing studies in most laboratories), which may also be responsible for hemolytic disease of the newborn. (d) Rubella antibody titers to document immune status. (e) Venereal disease research laboratories (VDRL) serology. **(2) Urine tests:** (a) Culture. (b) Biochemical urinalysis. **(3) Cervical swab:** (a) Culture. (b) Cytologic examination, if overdue.

Examination of the maternal abdomen follows the four classic **maneuvers of Leopold.** First, one determines which fetal parts are in the fundus by placing the examining hands on the uterine fundus while facing the mother's head. The hands are then passed along the sides of the uterus to determine on which side the fetal back lies. Next the right hand is placed just above the symphysis to determine the presentation by grasping the present-ing part between the thumb and forefinger. Rocking the presenting part back and forth indicates whether the presenting part has engaged (does not move freely). During the final maneuver the two hands are placed on either side of the lower portion of the uterine corpus while facing the patient's feet to determine on which side the cephalic prominence (provided the presentation is cephalic) is to be found permitting the diagnosis of fetal attitude.

Digital vaginal examination is usually deferred until the 3rd trimester *ct* when it can facilitate the diagnosis of position, station (distance, in cen-timeters above or below the ischial spines), and percentage effacement. The nongravid endocervical canal is 25 mm or 1 inch in length. Effacement refers to shortening of the endocervical canal during labor. Shortening by roughly 0.5 cm (0.25') represents 25% effacement.

A list of factors both medical and obstetric that qualify the **pregnancy as high risk** is given in Table 2-3. Patients with high risk pregnancies will require more frequent attention and perhaps referral to appropriate consultants.

A proposed outpatient visit schedule for normal pregnancies may be:

- q4wk until 28 weeks LMP
- q2wk from 28 to 36 weeks LMP
- weekly thereafter until delivery

Due to current western dietary mores many women of childbearing age are on the verge of iron deficiency anemia, their iron loss due to menses meeting or exceeding their iron intake. Iron supplements are therefore al-most routinely prescribed during pregnancy. Iron preparations should be administered after meals to diminish gastrointestinal irritation. Table 2-4 details the various forms of iron available pharmacologically. Note that plant sources of dietary iron are more often in the less well absorbed non-heme form, whereas animal sources are usually in the heme form. The usual dose is 300 mg ferrous sulfate daily or its equivalent. *300*

Anemia (macrocytic) may also result from inadequate folate intake and increased requirements (during both pregnancy and lactation). A multi-vitamin preparation containing folate (~5 mg/d) usually suffices.

**TABLE 2-3. FEATURES SUGGESTIVE OF HIGH-RISK PREGNANCY**

| Medical | Obstetric |
| --- | --- |
| Diabetes mellitus | Habitual spontaneous abortion |
| Thyroid disorders | Incompetent cervix |
| Cardiac disease | Maternal age: <17 yr; >35 yr |
| Hypertension | Prior cesarean section |
| Thromboembolic disease | Multiple gestation |
| Anemia | Prior fetal death |
| ITP | Preterm labor or SROM |
| Asthma | Uterine anomaly |
| Tuberculosis | Prior fetal anomalies |
| Renal disease | Rh Sensitization |
| Seizure disorder | Family history of heritable disease |
| Hepatitis | Small for gestational age |
| Obesity | |
| SLE | |
| Psychiatric disorder | |
| Syphilis | |

**ITP**, idiopathic thrombocytopenic purpura; **SROM**, spontaneous rupture of the membranes; **SLE**, systemic lupus erythematosus.

## Personal Comfort Items

Pregnancy, although a normal physiologic process, may be an uncomfortable 9 months. Several words are warranted with respect to avoiding or at least, making the best of certain inconveniences commonly encountered.

Mild laxatives and antacids are useful for constipation and dyspepsia respectively. Frequent small meals consisting of dry foods taken with ample fluid may diminish nausea and emesis. Hemorrhoidal discomfort can be alleviated somewhat by increased dietary fiber and stool softeners. The avoidance of agents with mild diuretic effects (caffeine, alcohol) will lessen any aggravation of bladder symptoms.

The discomfort of breast distension is minimized by proper support brassieres. In addition this may lessen undesirable cosmetic changes by diminishing the strain on Cooper's ligaments which support the breast.

TABLE 2-4. FORMS OF IRON AVAILABLE

| Preparation | Iron (%) | Elemental Iron (mg) | Iron/Salt Weight (mg) |
|---|---|---|---|
| Ferrous sulfate (FeSO$_4$ 7H$_2$O) | 20 | 60 | 300 |
| Exsciscated ferrous sulfate (FeSO$_4$ H$_2$O) | 33 | 66 | 200 |
| Ferrous lactate (Fe[C$_4$H$_2$O$_4$]$_2$) | 33 | 66 | 200 |
| Ferrous gluconate (Fe[C$_6$H$_{11}$O$_7$]$_2$) | 13 | 38 | 300 |

Moderate exercise is to be encouraged but strenuous activity can easily strain pelvic ligaments unnecessarily.

Normal clothing can be comfortably worn until obvious abdominal distension occurs at about the fourth month. At this time a switch to loose fitting garments that are supported from the shoulders becomes more reasonable. Support hosiery helps prevent the formation of varicosities. The prospective mother should also be advised to elevate her legs when reclining. High heels promote backache by exaggerating lumbar lordosis and should be avoided.

The **round ligament syndrome** refers to pelvic pain, usually right-sided (uterine dextrorotation) caused by stretching of the round ligament and relieved by laying decubitus with the offending flank dependent. Vaginal discharge or persistent spotting may make daily use of feminine napkins a necessity. Douches are to be proscribed and plain tub baths recommended.

Travel restrictions are unwarranted in an otherwise normal pregnancy. Sexual activity need not be curtailed for any medical reason and with some degree of creativity can continue until term.

## Notifiable Events

The patient should be instructed to report the occurrence of any of the following events to a physician: (1) any vaginal bleeding, especially if accompanied by pelvic cramps and (2) nonsteroidal anti-inflammatory drug (NSAID) refractory headaches, visual disturbances, oliguria, or excessive edema.

The onset of normal labor should be reviewed with the primigravid

*Labor = requires reg uc, cervical dilatation, effacement + Fetal descent*

patients. She should be instructed to get to hospital when regular low back or abdominal cramping occurs about every 4 to 5 minutes. Multiparous women should be advised to present as soon as regular pains commence. Both should be told to eat sparingly once they believe labor has commenced.

# LABOR

Labor is defined as the process by which the products of conception are separated and expelled from the uterus through the vagina. The clinical diagnosis of labor requires that regular uterine contractions, cervical dilatation, effacement and fetal descent occur. If this takes place before 37 weeks (LMP) gestational age, it is referred to as **preterm labor.** Eutocia refers to normal labor (cephalic presentation; no complications; the process is completed by the natural efforts of the mother). Dystocia refers to abnormal labor (deviation from any of the above criteria).

## Etiology

This is as yet unknown but numerous theories abound. The higher incidence of preterm labor in cases of polyhydramnios and multiple pregnancy provide circumstantial evidence that there exists a critical threshold for uterine volume, once exceeded it stimulates labor. Others suggest that pressure on the lower uterine segment and its nervous plexuses trigger labor. Placental senescence, by way of alterations in hormone production may be responsible. The fact that anencephalics (secondary hypoadrenalism) tend to deliver postterm and those with Cushing's syndrome (hypercortisolism) tend toward preterm delivery suggests that the fetal adrenal cortex may play a significant role in the onset of labor. It is clear, however, that adrenal steroids are not in themselves sufficient stimulus to induce labor. Furthermore they are often given without ill-effect when more expeditious labor is contraindicated, i.e., preterm labor.

## Three Stages of Labor

Classically labor is divided arbitrarily into three stages, however, there are processes that occur before true labor and shortly thereafter that also warrant mention.

TABLE 2-5. CLINICAL FEATURES OF LABOR

| True Labor | False Labor |
|---|---|
| ✱ **Pain** | |
| Progresses from back to front | Only anterior |
| Uterine firmness proportional to degree of discomfort | No relationship |
| Gradual increase in duration and severity | No change |
| Sedatives ineffective | Result in analgesia |
| **Pain Interval** | |
| Regular | Irregular |
| Gradually shortens | No change |
| **Presenting Part** | |
| Descends | No descent |
| Remains fixed between contractions | Remains free |
| Cervix effaced and dilated | Narrow cervical canal |

**Lightening,** the sensation of decreased abdominal distension that occurs 2 to 3 weeks before labor as the presenting part descends into the pelvis, is followed by **engagement** (the passage of the largest diameter of the presenting part through the pelvic inlet). Backache may become persistent, vaginal discharge may increase, and the cervical mucous plug may be extruded. There may also be a slight decline in body weight due to decreased water retention.

The clinical diagnosis of labor depends upon the characteristics of the pains accompanying uterine contractions, the time intervening between contractions, and progress of the fetal presenting parts (Table 2-5).

*First Stage.* **The first stage of labor commences with the onset of labor and ends with complete cervical dilatation (10 cm).** The duration of this stage is highly variable but is generally shorter in multiparous women, (2 to 10 hr) than in primigravidas (6 to 18 hr). Even before the onset of labor the **cervix ripens** (softens, shortens, and becomes dilatable). Relatively early in the course of pregnancy the cervix softens in consistency. In addition the cervix rotates anteriorly and the uterine corpus moves back so that their normal anteflexion and anteversion are corrected resulting in a straight path for the fetus during delivery. Dilatation of the cervical os to its maximum of 10 cm and effacement occur during this first stage of labor

*Effacement + dilatation*

The fetus floats in amniotic fluid surrounded by the amnion, which is itself enveloped by the chorion. As the cervix dilates, it abandons the membranes that precede the presenting part either tightly applied or as a palpable, fluctuant entity referred to as the **forewaters.**

The membranes usually do not rupture until the end of the second stage but when they do, contractions often become more efficient hastening the outcome of labor. It is not always apparent whether the membranes have indeed ruptured but circumstantial evidence includes: (1) seeing the escaping fluid either grossly or on speculum examination, (2) passage of meconium, and (3) alkaline vaginal pH as detected by nitrazine paper. The membranes, while intact, form a barrier to infection. Should they rupture without subsequent effective contractions, the risk of chorioamnionitis looms large. Spontaneous rupture of the membranes (SROM) is less likely to be followed by effective propulsive effort if it occurs prematurely (before the end of the second stage of term labor).

**Amniotomy** or artificial rupture of the membranes (ARM) is sometimes performed to stimulate labor. The risk of amnionitis becomes significant by about 24 hours after rupture; to avoid iatrogenic amnionitis ARM should not be performed until 3-cm cervical dilation is attained with the presenting part fixed in the pelvis and firmly applied to a ripe cervix thus ensuring that labor is well underway.

Passage of meconium with cephalic presentation may indicate fetal hypoxia, which promotes fetal intestinal peristalsis and sphincter laxity. Without concomitant suspicious fetal heart rate (FHR) changes this is not sufficient to justify immediate operative delivery. In the breech presentation meconium passage is attributed to simple mechanical compression of the bowels and is not a harbinger of impending demise.

Ecbolic maneuvers (those that stimulate myometrial contraction) include walking, coitus, enemas, nipple stimulation, amniotomy, and administration of oxytocic drugs. If both patients are healthy, the presentation is normal, and the presenting part engaged both walking and enemas can effectively shorten labor.

Frequent urination is encouraged to reduce the likelihood of bladder dystocia. Only clear fluids are permitted by mouth to prevent endobronchial aspiration should the mother become nauseated. An intravenous line may be

*IV*

indicated at this time for potential analgesic, oxytocic, or fluid administration. During this stage there is no benefit to be gained by bearing down with contractions and the mother should be advised to relax and conserve her energy. Sedatives may be indicated if she cannot manage this on her own. FHR should be checked fairly frequently (q15min) and pelvic examinations are performed routinely to ensure adequate progression.

*Second Stage.* **The second stage of labor is the interval between complete dilation of the cervix and delivery of the baby.** This takes anywhere from 1 to 3 hours in the primigravida but usually not in excess of 20 minutes for a multiparous woman. As the mother progresses to this stage, the discomfort with contractions intensifies and the latter become more frequent; she may want to bear down or defecate with the contractions and may become nauseated or retch.

The lithotomy position facilitates fetal monitoring, asepsis, and operative delivery but may promote supine hypotensive syndrome, endobronchial aspiration, and maternal discomfort. With the mother in a semi-Fowler's position (sitting up at 30-degree angle), many of these difficulties can be overcome and she can cooperate more effectively with each contraction.

Whereas bearing down during the first stage is counterproductive, it does hasten the termination of the second stage. Voluntary effort is facilitated by taking one or two deep breaths at the beginning of the contraction; holding the indrawn breath aids in fixing the diaphragm in place while pushing. As the presenting part **crowns** (passage of the largest diameter through the vulva) the introitus progresses from a narrow slit to a circular orifice. Crowning represents the "point of no return" as far as vaginal delivery is concerned and it also is the time when perineal lacerations are most likely.

A brief review of the mechanism of spontaneous delivery is in order. Left occiput anterior is the most common position. The six steps involved in delivery are (in order): **(1) descent; (2) flexion** of the head on the chest; **(3) internal rotation** of the head with respect to the maternal pelvis; **(4) extension** of the head at the neck with the nape anchored at the maternal symphysis (crowning); **(5) restitution** of the head back to the original LOA;

*Left occiput anterior*

*Crowning — time when perineal lacerations are most likely.*

then **(6) external rotation** of the entire body rendering the shoulders in the anteroposterior diameter. When the presentation is cephalic, the widest fetal diameter (occipitofrontal) passes through the pelvis first, usually dilating the maternal soft parts adequately to permit the body to slide out easily after the shoulders are delivered.

Controlled delivery of the head in the LOA position is the key to avoiding perineal damage. The goal here is to promote leisurely delivery of the head. Voluntary maternal assistance is discouraged at this point and the urge to push suppressed by panting to prevent fixation of the diaphragm. Usually events progress well on their own and all that is needed is gentle manual pressure on the fetal head to ensure controlled egress from the perineum.

On occasion delivery of the head is delayed prompting the accoucheur to perform one of the following maneuvers. The **Ritgen procedure** consists of fundal pressure on the head as the occiput rests at the symphisis while the other hand presses per rectum to encourage extension of the chin. Alternately the fingers may be passed per vaginum by the cheek and around the chin, which is "hooked out" over the perineum. If the orifice appears to be insufficiently large and laceration imminent, an episiotomy may be performed. The direction and length of the incision can be controlled obviating difficult perineal repairs.

Immediately after the head delivers by extension it is supported as it restitutes and externally rotates; the airways are suctioned of mucus and the neck is explored for possible umbilical cord. If the cord is wound around the neck it may be loose enough to be unwrapped; however, if this is not possible simply double clamp the cord, cut, then unwrap. With hands over the face and the occiput, the head is depressed then elevated to assist delivery of the anterior and posterior shoulders, respectively. Traction should not be applied on the head, this may lead to brachial plexus damage (**Erb-Duchenne palsy**). The baby is held face down with the third and fourth fingers straddling the neck, the body supported by the forearm and a leg secured between the forearm and the accoucheur's trunk. If not already done, the cord is now doubly clamped and cut.

Should neonatal resuscitation be necessary, airway suctioning and oxygen by mask prove successful in the vast majority. If the baby is persistently unresponsive the airway should be suctioned under direct laryngoscopic

Erb-Duchenne Palsy

visualization before the institution of positive pressure (bag-and-mask) ventilation to prevent meconium aspiration. After an adequate airway is secured, cardiac massage (120 to 140 compressions per minute) and intravenous NaHCO$_3$ are administered as necessary (see section on Neonatal Assessment).

*Third Stage.* **The third stage of labor commences after the delivery of the baby and terminates when the placenta is delivered.** It is generally 5 to 20 minutes in duration. The initial phase of placental expulsion starts within 5 minutes of the termination of the second stage. It is characterized by a gush of vaginal blood with lengthening of the cord outside the vulva as a firm globular fundus rises in the abdomen. Separation is aided either by voluntary effort or gentle fundal pressure. The placenta is examined to ensure that it is complete. Retained remnants promote both postpartum hemorrhage and infection. Delayed placental separation may result from: (1) failure to separate; (2) **placenta accreta** (deficient decidua permitting chorionic villi to penetrate into the myometrium); or (3) a separated placenta retained by an abnormally spastic cervix. Manual exploration of the uterus is indicated if (1) placental examination is suggestive of retained fragments, (2) placenta not delivered in 30 minutes without hemorrhage, (3) immediately if hemorrhage is significant, and (4) after traumatic delivery to detect possible lacerations. Notwithstanding, the cervix, vagina, and perineum must always be examined for lacerations.

For the first hour after labor is completed the mother must be observed closely for signs of hemorrhage (doughy uterus, vaginal bleeding, inappropriate vital signs) and the infant should be examined to ensure adequate cardiorespiratory function and the absence of major malformations.

## NEONATAL ASSESSMENT

The immediate assessment of the newborn infant requires a knowledge of the events of (1) gestation (duration, hemorrhage, hypertension, infections); (2) labor (duration, relative timing of rupture of membranes, anesthesia); and (3) delivery (fetal presentation, surgical interventions, fetal anomalies).

The physical examination pays particular attention to the car-

Asphyxia =

**TABLE 2-6. ASPHYXIA AND ITS PREVENTION**

| Prerequisites for Normal Gas Exchange | Potential Disorders Leading to Asphyxia |
|---|---|
| **Antenatal** | |
| Normal maternal $PaO_2$ | Maternal cardiorespiratory diseases; excessive sedation |
| Healthy, firmly attached placenta | PIH; placenta previa; abruptio placentae |
| Unobstructed umbilical vascular flow | Prolapsed, knotted, or ruptured cord; prolonged labor |
| **Postnatal** | |
| Functional neonatal CNS respiratory center | Excessive sedation; intracranial hemorrhage |
| Healthy neonatal heart and lungs | Congenital heart disease; congenital lung disease; diaphragmatic (**Bochdalek**) hernia |
| Airway patency | Aspiration (meconium, mucous, blood); **micrognathia**; choanal atresia |

diorespiratory status of the neonatal patient to detect possible asphyxia. **Asphyxia** is defined as the actual or apparent cessation of life due to an interruption of gaseous exchange in the lungs. A list of the antenatal and postnatal prerequisites for the avoidance of asphyxia, as well as the possible disorders leading to asphyxia, are given in Table 2-6.

Antenatally, asphyxia is most accurately detected by sampling venous blood for blood gas analysis. More commonly, however, it is detected by fetal heart rate monitoring (late or variable decelerations) or the observation of meconium in the liquid (cephalic presentation).

Postnatally a standardized set of observations of cardiorespiratory and basic neurologic function (**APGAR scoring**) is used to provide an overall score that indicates the severity of neonatal asphyxia. This scoring system yields reproducible results. The patient is assessed at 1 and 5 minutes postpartum (the latter bears more prognostic information) (Table 2-7).

Resuscitative efforts to be undertaken are guided by the APGAR score (Table 2-8).

Prolonged asphyxia leads to circulatory failure (''shock''). Thus if the infant survives, renal and gut function must be closely monitored. Cerebral

**TABLE 2-7. APGAR SCORING**   *To assess neonatal asphyxia*

| | Score | | |
|---|---|---|---|
| | **0** | **1** | **2** |
| Appearance | Blue | Blue/pink | Pink |
| Pulse | Absent | <100/min | >100/min |
| Grimace (stimulus response) | Absent | Grimaces | Cough/sneeze |
| Activity (muscle tone) | Flaccid | Flexed extremities | Active motion |
| Respiratory effort | Absent | Weak/irregular | Crying with vigor |
| **Total Score** | **Degree of Asphyxia** | | **Prognosis** |
| 0–3 | Severe | | Moribund |
| 4–6 | Moderate | | Variable |
| >7 | None | | Normal |

(seizure disorder, mental retardation, cerebral palsy) and cardiorespiratory (congestive heart failure due to global ischemia, respiratory distress syndrome) dysfunction may follow severe or prolonged asphyxia.

Once time permits a more complete physical examination can be undertaken (see next page).

**TABLE 2-8. NEONATAL RESUSCITATION**

| General Sequence | APGAR Scores and Specific Procedures Indicated | | |
|---|---|---|---|
| | **APGAR >7** | **APGAR 4–6** | **APGAR <4** |
| **Assure airway patency** | Inspect oropharynx with naked eye | | Laryngoscopic examination |
| **Stimulate** | Tap hands and feet | | Omit |
| **Ventilate** | Bag and mask, +/− ETI | | Immediate ETI |
| **"Circulate"** | Omit | Omit | External cardiac compression and umbilical catheterization |
| **Warm** | Dry infant and place under heater | | |

**ETI**, endotracheal intubation.

- *Vital signs:* Apical heart rate; respiratory rate.
- *Appearance:* Vigor of cry and skin color; obvious anomalies.
- *Respiratory:* Visible respiratory effort; "grunting"; percussion (for possible pneumothorax); breath sounds.
- *Cardiac:* Auscultation (extra heart sounds or murmurs); thrills/ heaves; adequacy of femoral pulses.
- *Remainder of vital signs:* Temperature; weight; height; head circumference; blood pressure.
- *Abdomen:* Contour; masses (hepatosplenomegaly, enlarged kidneys); bowel sounds; anal patency; umbilicus (three vessels).
- *Skin:* Hematomas; edema.
- *Head:* Molding; caput succadeneum; cephalohematoma; fontanels; integrity of lips, gums, and palate; suck reflex; epicanthic folds (prominence suggestive of dysmorphism); strabismus; pinnae.
- ⊙*Neck:* Rigidity; "webbing"; trachea midline.
- *Genitourinary:* External genitalia of one sex only; testicular descent in male.
- ⊙*Extremities:* Clavicular integrity; Ortolani test (especially female infants); appropriate number and form of digits.
- *Neurologic:* Moro reflex; grasp reflex; rooting reflex; Deep Tendon Reflex (DTRs); motor activity of all appendages; response to noxious stimulus.

## PUERPERIUM   First 6 wks Postpartum

The term puerperium is defined as the period of confinement during and immediately after delivery. By convention the puerperium includes the first 6 weeks postpartum. During this interval the genitourinary tract and the hypothalamic–pituitary–gonadal axis return to the nonpregnant state (except for some permanent changes) and the breasts initiate lactation.

The 1-kg postpartal uterus involutes by means of cell shrinkage rather than cell loss and within 1 week it weighs 500 g, 100 g at 2 weeks, and returns to normal by 4 weeks. The superficial layer of endometrium beyond the placental bed sloughs, while the deep basalis layer regenerates a normal surface. The placental bed differs because it is composed of many throm-

uterus size returns to nl w/in 4 wks

*Colostrum - 2-5d post partum. Protein / mineral*
*rich but lipid / CH₂O poor initial form*
*of milk.*

NORMAL OBSTETRICS    **39**

bosed vessels that, if allowed to organize normally, would form a scar. Progressive endometrial cicatrization would thus limit ultimate reproductive ✓ capacity. This is prevented by sloughing of the placental bed with ingrowth of the adjacent endometrium to fill the gap.

The floppy, distensible postpartal cervix and lower uterine segment may continue to admit up to two fingers for the first week but thereafter they regain their usual consistency. The external os is, however, permanently altered with (usually) lateral clefting due to lacerations sustained during delivery. Although the vaginal lumen remains permanently enlarged, the rugae return within 3 weeks.

Menses recur in 6 to 8 weeks if nonlactating and in 2 to 18 months in lactating women. It is thought that lactation results in lowered gonadotropin levels thus leading to amenorrhea. Nonetheless it is often difficult to ascertain the exact time of resumption of menses due to ongoing vaginal discharge. Contraception should be reinstituted early (3 weeks postpartum) unless immediate repeat pregnancy is to be hazarded.

The capacity of the urinary bladder is increased and its sensitivity to distension decreased during pregnancy, thus predisposing to stasis and infection. Furthermore the dilated renal drainage system increases the chances of upward progression of lower tract infections. *More common on (R)*

From day 2 to 5 postpartum the breasts become engorged and exude **colostrum,** which is the protein/mineral-rich but lipid/carbohydrate-poor initial form of milk. In addition to the nutrient value of human milk there are also protective immunologic factors transferred from mother to infant (**IgA** may protect against enteric infection; **lysozyme** may inactivate gram-positive micorbes; **lactoferrin** may chelate iron in the gut making it unavailable to iron-dependent bacteria).

Complex, poorly understood mechanisms underlie the onset of milk formation. The rapid decline in female sex steroids incumbent upon loss of the placenta is thought to play a significant role and although prolactin (prerequisite for lactation) levels also fall after delivery of the placenta the suckling-induced elevations of this hormone are believed to be sufficient to maintain milk production. Suckling also stimulates the neurohypophysis to secrete oxytocin causing contraction of the breast myoepithelial cells that surround the milk-producing acini thus expelling milk.

*Mastitis = S. aureus / S. epidermis treat c̄ nafcillin / dicloxacillin.*

# Clinical

*milk fever*

A slight rise in temperature occasionally accompanies the initiation of lactation. Because of the substantial risk of infection during puerperium, however, any temperature in excess of 38.0C occurring after the first 24 hours should be investigated fully with appropriate cultures. Possible sites of infection include: (1) genital tract (episiotomy site, endometritis); (2) urinary tract (cystitis, pyelonephritis); and (3) breasts (mastitis). Infections not specific to the puerperium may also cause fever, e.g., respiratory or intravenous catheter phlebitis. The causative organisms of both the genital and urinary infections are usually gram-negative bacilli that respond to the usual antibiotics (e.g., ampicillin, aminoglycosides). Mastitis is usually the result of a *Staphylococcus aureus* infection, requiring a penicillinase-resistant synthetic penicillin (e.g., cloxacillin, nafcillin).

**Afterpains** refer to the persistent irregular occurrence of uncomfortable uterine contractions after delivery. This discomfort is exacerbated by the suckling-induced release of oxytocin that promotes myometrial contraction. Afterpains generally abate within 3 to 4 days.

**Lochia** is the term applied to puerperal vaginal discharge. Lochia is initially (3 to 4 days) red (**lochia rubra**) due to the admixture of endometrial slough containing red blood cells but lightens progressively (**lochia serosa,** day 4 to 10; **lochia alba,** day 10 on) as the leukocytic content becomes predominant.

*5th*

A postpartum diuresis usually occurs by the fifth day due to a reversal of the fluid retaining hormonal influences of pregnancy. Ketonuria is not uncommon immediately after prolonged labor and is attributable to starvation. Apparent glycosuria is usually due to excessive lactose production at the breast.

*WBC ↑*

*ESR*

Leukocytosis, up to 30,000 × $10^3$/L predominantly polymorphonuclear leukocytes (PMN), is common and, therefore, not helpful in implicating an ongoing infectious process. The erythrocyte sedimentation rate (ESR) elevation characteristic of pregnancy persists for a week or two. Concurrent extracellular fluid (ECF) volume losses effectively compensate for red blood cell loss, so that the Hb level rarely falls by more than 10 g/L unless substantial hemorrhage has occurred.

There is an overall weight loss of ~7 kg due to the expulsion of the fetus and other uterine contents (5 kg) and the fluid loss by diuresis (2 kg).

## Management

Immediately after delivery the uterine fundus should be examined several times to ensure that it remains firm and does not increase in size suggesting internal bleeding. The perineum should be rinsed with soapy water, directing the fluid from the mons to the anus and a sterile pad applied. The pad should be checked regularly for evidence of bleeding.

Oral narcotic analgesics and topical perineal sprays are indicated for the many causes (episiotomy, laceration, breast engorgement, spinal puncture) of puerperal pain. If these agents prove inadequate, careful perineal and speculum examination to exclude hematoma formation is indicated. Episiotomies are generally healed and asymptomatic within 3 weeks.

Urinary retention is suggested if the patient has not voided within 4 hours of delivery. Persistent anesthetic blockade and local pain may be responsible. Light ambulation should be attempted before one resorts to catheterization.

For those who deliver vaginally a normal diet is permissible after 2 uncomplicated hours have elapsed since delivery. Ambulation (assisted initially to avoid syncopal injury) within 24 hours of delivery reduces the incidence of thromboembolism, urinary retention, and constipation. Abdominal wall exercises to diminish laxity can be commenced the day of delivery.

The nipples should be kept clean of excess milk to avoid fissuring and infection. If the former occurs, nipple shields can be used for 24 hours. Nursing bras that support but do not constrict are prudent during the puerperium. Not uncommonly the initial volume of milk produced is disappointing and frustrating, especially due to uncomfortable engorgement. The mother should be reassured and supported during this interval until milk flow becomes properly established. If, however, the mother chooses not to nurse, bromocriptine, 2.5 mg PO BID for 2 weeks, will halt further milk production.

The physical discomforts of the puerperium, fatigue and postanticipatory sadness, characteristic of any emotional denouement in addition to anxieties concerning body image and the attendant responsibilities of motherhood often combine to make the new mother quite dysphoric. Mutual reassurance and support between the new parents (facilitated by advance warning of the likelihood of such apprehensions) obviates physician inter-

*Bromocryptine 2.5 mg*
*PO BID X 14 d*
*DA agonist*

vention. Occasionally this episode may unmask a clinical depressive illness.

Discharge home is usually not delayed beyond the third day postpartum. Rh immunoglobulin and rubella immunization are administered before discharge where indicated. Although the mother can resume normal bathing, driving, and occupational activities upon discharge, the resumption of the latter are often delayed by infant care especially in the first-time mother. The only hindrance to the resumption of sexual activity is possible dyspareunia. A follow-up visit between 3 and 6 weeks postpartum permits detection of any late postpartal problems and the institution of contraception.

# 3

# Abnormal Obstetrics

## VAGINAL BLEEDING AND PREGNANCY

This discussion is presented in three parts: vaginal bleeding during the first 20 weeks of gestation (Table 3-1), vaginal bleeding during the second 20 weeks of gestation (Table 3-2), and postpartum hemorrhage (PPH). The latter section is further broken down into early and late PPH.

Vaginal bleeding during pregnancy may range in significance from trivial to life-threatening for both fetus and mother. The source of the bleeding is either maternal or fetoplacental. The former is more common. Maternal sources for vaginal bleeding during pregnancy can be viewed as arising from the upper (fallopian tubes or corpus uteri) or the lower (uterine cervix, vagina, or vulva) genitourinary tract. Lower tract sources, particularly cervical lesions are much more common. So much so that the presence of a cervical lesion should not halt investigation for a possible coexisting upper tract lesion, which may be of much greater significance.

Upper genitourinary tract lesions include: (1) decidual breakdown due to loss of hormonal (progestational) support; (2) placental separation (this represents the early pregnancy counterpart to abruptio placentae) with hemorrhage from the subplacental venous sinuses; and (3) spontaneous abortion, the loss of a potentially normal intrauterine fetus (most occur during the first 6 to 10 weeks of gestation and up to 20% have marked chromosomal aberrations). Two forms of fundamentally abnormal pregnancy are also potential causes of upper tract bleeding: extrauterine or ectopic pregnancy and hydatidiform mole. Both of these entities are discussed in separate sections of the notes.

43

**TABLE 3-1. VAGINAL BLEEDING DURING THE FIRST 20 WEEKS OF GESTATION**

| Cause | Clinical Information | Uterine Size | Investigations | Treatment |
|---|---|---|---|---|
| Blighted ovum | Late period; +/− transient evidence of pregnancy | Prepregnant | Review menstrual history; U/S | D & C |
| Cervical lesion | Postcoital bleeding; bleeding lesion visible on inspection | AGA | Pap smear; biopsy if necessary; U/S normal for gestation | Dependent on the nature of disease; not altered by pregnancy |
| Threatened abortion[a] | No cervical lesion; light bleed; no uterine contractions; cervical os closed | AGA | Serum beta-HCG remains positive; U/S normal for gestation | Observe; cervical cerclage if cervix incompetent |
| Incomplete abortion | Heavy bleed; clots +/− conceptus; uterine contractions; open os; bleeding may taper spontaneously | AGA/SGA | Serum beta-HCG useful if reverts to negative; U/S absence of gestational sac | Crystalloid resuscitation; ecbolic agents; D & C to remove nidus for infection; anticipate sepsis |
| Missed abortion[b] | Regression of amenorrhea, nausea/emesis, bladder irritability, breast heaviness | Fails to enlarge over a significant time interval | Serum beta-HCG negative; U/S abnormal | Evacuate remnants; anticipate DIC if >4 wk |
| GTD | (See separate discussion) | | | |

[a]All vaginal bleeding during pregnancy should be regarded as threatened abortion until proven otherwise.
[b]Dead fetus that has not yet been expelled.
AGA, appropriate for gestational age; D & C, dilatation and curettage; DIC, disseminated intravascular coagulation; GTD, Gestational Trophoblastic disease; SGA, small for gestational age; U/S, ultrasound.

Lower genitourinary tract lesions, specifically cervical lesions include:
(1) cervical eversion of pregnancy, (2) benign polyps, and (3) carcinoma of
the cervix.

## Management of Placenta Previa

The initial hemorrhage is often self-limited and serves to herald a second
more serious event. The fetus is often immature, therefore the goal of
therapy is to prolong gestation by preventing serious hemorrhage. The patient should be admitted and four units of cross-matched blood should be
available for the patient at all times. Amniocentesis may be performed to
determine the lecithin/sphingomyelin (L/S) ratio (see section on preterm
labor). Once the diagnosis is established by ultrasound (U/S), digital vaginal
examination should be avoided because it may trigger precipitous bleeding.

Once the pregnancy has reached 37 weeks last menstrual period (LMP)
with fetal pulmonary maturity or if the bleeding is profuse, pregnancy must
be terminated. It is almost always preferable to perform a cesarean section
especially if: on U/S the placenta is seen to be a total previa or a partial
previa covering more than 10% of the cervical os; bleeding is profuse; there
is evidence of fetal distress; or the presentation is abnormal. Some authorities suggest that if: the bleed is minimal, the presentation is cephalic,
the head is engaged, the cervix is at least 3 cm dilated, and the placenta
overlies less than 10% of the orifice of the os, then a trial of induction is
permissible.     *TOL*

## Management of Abruptio Placentae

Crystalloid resucitation by a wide bore intravenous catheter followed by
transfusion of blood products as soon as they become available are immediately indicated in the setting of acute circulatory failure. Prompt delivery of
the fetus is advisable for the benefit of both maternal and fetal welfare. This
acts to decrease the likelihood of disseminated intravascular coagulation
(DIC) in the mother as well as fetal mortality, which is proportional to the
length of the time interval between onset of hemorrhage and delivery.

In most circumstances cesarean section is the mode of delivery of
choice when the fetus is alive. It is also indicated if the fetus is dead but
hemorrhage is uncontrolled. Delivery by induced labor can be attempted in a

**TABLE 3-2. VAGINAL BLEEDING DURING THE SECOND 20 WEEKS OF GESTATION**

| Cause | Clinical | Investigations | Associated Conditions |
|---|---|---|---|
| **Placenta previa** (the placenta lies on or near the internal cervical os in advance of the presenting part; may be total, partial, or marginal) | **Painless** vaginal bleed; initial bleed often self-limiting; uterus **soft/nontender**; FHR **present**; presenting part high; degree of hypovolemia **proportional to** visible bleed | Do **not** perform digital pelvic examination; U/S most safe and accurate; soft tissue X-ray of pelvis | May reflect decidual insufficiency in upper uterine segment requiring placenta to spread over greater surface; failed engagement; abnormal presentations; congenital anomalies; placenta accreta; PPH |
| **Abruptio placentae** (premature separation of the placenta with bleed into decidua basalis then; enters amniotic fluid or tracks down to cervix and vagina; may be total or partial) | **Painful** bleed; with internal bleeds degree of hypovolemia **exceeds** amount of visible bleed; uterus **firm and tender;** FHR **absent;** may be less painful with external bleed | CBC, Plt; PT/PTT; fibrinogen; U/S | Hypertensive disorders of pregnancy; uterine overdistension; fetal trauma; short umbilical cord |

a or tracks down to

| | | | | |
|---|---|---|---|---|
| **Vasa previa** (presentation of the fetal vessels across internal cervical os) | Bleed due to tearing of fetal vessels; marked fetal bradycardia during uterine contraction due to vessel compression; vessels may be palpable on pelvic examination | Dx rarely apparent before labor; **Kleihauer test of vaginal blood to detect fetal RBCs**; pelvic examination (60% fetal mortality) | | Low-lying placenta; velamentous insertion of the cord[b] |
| **Rupture of the marginal sinus** (vascular channel that rims the placenta returning blood to maternal circulation) | Light, painless bleed | None usually required (+/− U/S) | Nil | |

[a]Couvelaire uterus.

[b]Umbilical cord inserts into the membranes with vessels running between the amnion and the chorion.

**CBC**, complete blood count; **Dx**, diagnosis; **FRH**, fetal heart rate; **Plt**, platelet; **PPH**, postpartum hemorrhage; **PT/PTT**, Prothrombin Time partial thromboplastin time; **RBC**, red blood cell; **U/S**, ultrasound.

Note: Maternal mortality with abruptio placentae is < 1% but fetal mortality may approach 50%. For placenta previa, fetal mortality is ~15%.

$C-Hy s$

multiparous woman if the cervix is 3 cm dilated and the head is deep in the pelvis. Should hemorrhage continue despite delivery of the fetus, hysterectomy is indicated.

Complications that can arise include: (1) DIC, (2) PPH, (3) acute renal failure due to hypovolemia or DIC, or both, and (4) **Sheehan's syndrome.** The latter refers to adenohypophyseal necrosis thought to result from circulatory insufficiency. This manifests subsequently as panhypopituitarism.

## Management of Vasa Previa

Vasa previa represents one of the instances of primarily fetal blood loss. If bleeding is the mode of presentation, either cesarean or vaginal delivery should be carried out at once. If the prolapsing fetal vessels are detected by palpation without hemorrhage at full dilatation, amniotomy and vaginal delivery can be undertaken, otherwise cesarean section should be considered. Blood transfusion for the infant is usually required once delivered. In the event that the fetus has died in utero, it is acceptable to await spontaneous vaginal delivery.

## Management of Rupture of the Marginal Sinus

Rupture of the marginal sinus is a normal event at the end of the second stage of delivery but it may occur during the late third trimester. Little needs to be done usually because fetal distress rarely occurs and the magnitude of the hemorrhage is rarely significant.

## Idiopathic

If bleeding occurs in the third trimester and it cannot be assigned to any of the above processes and no cervical lesion is found, only observation and supportive care can be offered until the bleed ceases or declares itself.

## Postpartum Hemorrhage

Postpartum hemorrhage is defined as any vaginal blood loss after the second stage of labor that exceeds 500 ml (Tables 3-3 and 3-4).

*Early Postpartum Hemorrhage.* Early postpartum hemorrhage refers to any postpartum hemorrhage occurring within 24 hours of delivery. It is

### TABLE 3-3. PREDISPOSING CONDITIONS

*Uterine Overdistension*
Multiple pregnancy
Polyhydramnios
Prolonged Labor
Grand multipara

*Operative Delivery*
Cesarean section
Difficult forceps delivery
Deep anesthesia

*Third Trimester Hemorrhage*
Placenta previa
Abruptio placentae

*Other*
Prior history
Missed abortion

*3rd space losses*

$$nl = 250 \, mL$$

stated that normal delivery may involve up to 250-ml of blood loss. The expanded extracellular fluid (ECF) volume characteristic of pregnancy can permit as much as a 500-ml blood loss without serious hemodynamic consequences. Hemorrhage into the uterus represents a "third space" or ineffective extravascular extracellular fluid (EVECF) volume loss, which may result in acute circulatory failure with relatively little external evidence of blood.

The chief complications of PPH are postpartum infection and death. Death due to PPH is almost never immediate suggesting it should be preventable provided appropriate resuscitative measures are undertaken.

### TABLE 3-4. MECHANISMS OF PPH

Uterine atony *90%*
Lacerations and trauma
Retained placenta
Bleeding diathesis

*Uterine Atony.* Postpartum control of uterine hemorrhage is affected by contraction and retraction of myometrial fibers causing kinking of the intramural vasculature. If this mechanism fails then there will be excessive blood loss at the site of placental separation.

In addition to the listed predisposing conditions both leiomyomata and ineffective uterine action during the first two stages of labor increase the likelihood of uterine atony.

Management of PPH due to uterine atony may involve uterine massage, ecbolic agents, manual uterine exploration (and removal of blood clots or retained fragments of placenta), and compression of the aorta. Uterine packing is a controversial issue. Most obstetricians believe that it merely prevents the myometrial fibers from contracting properly, exacerbating the blood loss. Should these measures be unsuccessful, operative intervention becomes mandatory. A vascular surgeon may be consulted to ligate the internal iliac arteries thereby limiting the major source of blood flow. The profuse collateral system of the pelvis prevents necrosis of pelvic organs from occurring. Note that the vessels are only ligated and not transected thus permitting the later possibility of recanalization. Should all other measures prove unsuccessful, hysterectomy becomes the method of last resort, sacrificing subsequent fertility.

*Lacerations & Trauma.* When the vulva does not stretch sufficiently as the fetal head is crowning, the risk of laceration is increased with subsequent hemorrhage. Operative deliveries and any delivery involving an episiotomy also runs the added risk of hemorrhage from local sites of injury. Thus with every delivery the cervix, vagina, and perineum must be inspected for evidence of trauma. Any bleeding vessels encountered during such inspection should be clamped immediately and then ligated. Note that rupture of the uterus usually represents upward extension of a cervical laceration, thus a high index of suspicion must be maintained when the latter is found. Excessive traction of the placenta during the third stage of labor may result in uterine inversion (prolapse of uterine apex through the cervix), which promotes bleeding. Occasionally bleeding is retained locally in the immediate postpartum situation only to present as a puerperal hematoma that ruptures and bleeds at a later date.

Lacerations or trauma, limited to the perineum, are usually adequately managed by oversewing with figure-of-eight sutures. Sites of vaginal bleeding may be managed by packing with gauze for 24 hours. Uterine rupture necessitates emergent laparotomy and repair or resection (i.e., hysterectomy).

**Retained Placenta.** In general anything within the postpartum uterus will prevent proper contraction and retraction of the myometrium thus resulting in secondary uterine atony. The endometrium at the site of an incompletely separated placenta will therefore continue to bleed. There is no correlation between the amount of tissue retained and the severity of the bleed.

Whenever this condition is suspect (placenta delivered is noted to be incomplete on inspection), manual exploration of the uterus is indicated. Extraction of the retained fragments will lead to cessation of the hemorrhage.

**Bleeding Diathesis.** Pregnant women may experience any of the known hemorrhagic diseases that can occur in nonpregnant women, but in addition to these they are at increased risk of DIC and amniotic fluid embolism.

**Disseminated intravascular coagulation** may complicate fetal death especially if the fetus is not promptly expelled from the uterus (Table 3-5). DIC is a syndrome that occurs when normal coagulation factors, are consumed by abnormal activation of the clotting system. DIC usually presents as a bleeding diathesis with bleeding from needle puncture sites, ecchymoses, and hematomas. All laboratory clotting studies are affected, however, the platelet count is most sensitive and slowest to return to normal. Management includes correcting the underlying problem and supportive hematologic measures (Table 3-6).

**TABLE 3-5. OBSTETRIC PROBLEMS ASSOCIATED WITH DIC**

Abruptio placentae
Fetal death
Amniotic fluid embolism
Septic or saline abortion
Pregnancy-induced hypertension

**TABLE 3-6. MANAGEMENT OF DIC**

| Laboratory Tests | Management |
|---|---|
| ↓ Fibrinogen | |
| ↑ Prothrombin time (PT) | Delivery of fetus and fresh |
| ↑ Partial thromboplastin time (PTT) | frozen plasma (FFP) |
| ↑ Thrombin time (TT) | |
| ↑ Fibrin(ogen) degradation products (FDP) | |
| ↓ Platelets | Transfuse platelets |
| ↓ Hemoglobin | Transfuse packed RBCs |
| Fragmented RBCs on peripheral smear | |

**Amniotic fluid embolism** is a relatively rare event (1/2000 pregnancies) associated with: (1) rapid labor in multiparous patients and (2) operative (forceps) deliveries. It presents with rapid onset of cardiovascular collapse and DIC (hemorrhage). As better methods of dealing with obstetric complications have evolved this condition has assumed a more important place as a significant cause of maternal morbidity and mortality.

*Late Postpartum Hemorrhage.* As noted previously this is defined as a vaginal blood loss in excess of 500 ml occurring more than 24 hours, but less than 42 days postpartum. Possible causes of late postpartum hemorrhage include:

Uterine
    Retained placenta
    Endometritis
    Uterine subinvolution
    Large submucosal myoma
    Early estrogen therapy
Extrauterine
    Cervicitis
    Vaginitis
    Vulvar cellulitis

Infection, whether intrauterine or extrauterine acts to promote dissolution of thrombi and sloughing of the overlying layers of tissues (as well as sutures) that are responsible for maintaining hemostasis at sites of injury. Management consists of local debridement (with or without repeat suturing, depending on the appearance at the time) and pressure dressings.

Mechanisms postulated for late uterine PPH include: late detachment of thrombi, abnormal decidual separation, and infection (as described previously). Management consists of ecbolic agents, dilatation and curettage (D & C), antibiotics if necessary, and perhaps repeat D & C or even hysterectomy.

## PREGNANCY-INDUCED HYPERTENSION

Pregnancy-induced hypertension (PIH) represents one of the triad of major complications of pregnancy (the others being hemorrhage and sepsis). The existence of hypertension in pregnancy is defined as either (1) an increase in the systolic pressure of > 30 mmHg or an increase in the diastolic of > 15 mmHg or (2) a blood pressure > 140/90 on two occasions more than 6 hours apart.

**Pregnancy-induced hypertension** formerly referred to as **pre-eclampsia** is defined as the trial of hypertension, edema, and proteinuria, usually after 20 weeks LMP, frequently near term. The presence of the triad before 20 weeks LMP is suggestive of molar pregnancy. **Eclampsia** refers to preeclampsia complicated by seizure activity in a patient with no prior history of seizure disorder.

Proteinuria in pregnancy is defined as (1) urine protein concentration > 0.3 g/L in a 24-hour sample or (2) urine protein concentration > 1.0 g/L in random urine samples on at least two separate occasions. Edema refers to excess extravascular extracellular fluid (EVECF) and is most apparent at the eyelids, hands, and ankles.

Blood pressure (BP) varies predictably during normal pregnancy. BP normally falls slightly during the first two trimesters with a subsequent return to nonpregnant levels during the third trimester. The upper limit of normal for diastolic pressures during the first two trimesters is 75 to 80 mmHg and 85 to 90 mmHg for the third trimester. Values in excess of these limits are consistent with a diagnosis of hypertension in pregnancy. During the first two trimesters BPs, which could be interpreted as only slightly

*PIH 5-10% in general OB pop.*
*① intravascular extracellular vol depletion*
*② systemic vasoconstriction*

elevated by nonpregnant standards, may in fact be indicative of significant hypertension.

**Coincident hypertension and pregnancy (CHP),** formerly chronic hypertension, is defined as the presence of persistent hypertension regardless of cause before 20 weeks LMP gestation in the absence of gestational trophoblastic disease or BP elevation continuing for > 6 months after delivery. PIH can also be superimposed on coincident hypertension and this is best detected by the first definition provided for hypertension in pregnancy.

*Epidemiology.* The incidence of PIH is 5% to 10% among the general obstetrical population but as high as 25% in the population with preexistant hypertension. Patients at risk for PIH often have the features listed in Table 3-7. The incidence of PIH may be overestimated because of the difficulty in diagnosing coincident hypertension antedating pregnancy in a patient seen for the first time during the first trimester. Perinatal mortality may reach 30%, whereas maternal mortality is < 10%. Up to 25% of patients may have recurrent PIH, especially those with pregnancy-aggravated hypertension (Table 3-7). Although not proven, it may be that patients with PIH are at

---

**TABLE 3-7. CLASSIFICATION OF HYPERTENSION AND PREGNANCY**

*Pregnancy-induced hypertension*
1. Edema and proteinuria **absent**
   Mild
   Severe[a]
2. Edema and proteinuria **present** (preeclampsia)
   Mild
   Severe[a]
3. Edema, proteinuria, and **convulsions** (eclampsia)

*Coincident hypertension*
1. Pregnancy-unaltered hypertension
2. Pregnancy-aggravated hypertension
   Superimposed preeclampsia
   Superimposed eclampsia

---

[a]Blood pressure in excess of 160/110, heavy proteinuria with occasional liver failure and coagulopathy resembling DIC.

increased risk for subsequent development of hypertension while not ✓ pregnant.

Although pregnancy may not affect coincident hypertension the high blood pressure does pose risk for both the fetus (abruptio placenta, intrauterine growth retardation, midtrimester death) and the mother (acute renal failure, cerebral hemorrhage). Coincident hypertension due to pheochromocytoma or Cushing's syndrome is associated with particularly poor maternal and fetal outcome. Predictors of poor fetal outcome include maternal age >30 years and prolonged duration of hypertension before pregnancy. Pregnancy-aggravated hypertension has the highest morbidity and mortality rates for both mother and child (Table 3-8).

*Pathophysiology.* The etiology of PIH is unknown. Several hypotheses have been promulgated including uteroplacental insufficiency, an immunologic reaction to the chorionic villi, and even a definite autosomal recessive heritable factor. None of these theories alone provides an adequate explanation of the cause for this disease.

Although controversy abounds, there is universal agreement that PIH is characterized by: (1) intravascular extracellular fluid (IVECF) volume depletion and (2) systemic vasoconstriction. Unfortunately this is where agreement ends. Certain authorities suggest that the decline in the IVECF volume is the primary event with secondary vasoconstriction (perhaps related to decreased uterine $PGE_2$ or PGI synthesis), whereas others feel that vasospasm is the primary event with IVECF volume depletion being secondary.

**TABLE 3-8. EPIDEMIOLOGIC RISK FACTORS FOR PIH**

Hypertension antedating pregnancy
Low maternal age    $< 17$
Multiple pregnancy
Positive family history (first degree relatives)
✳ Primigravida
Short stature (maternal) ?
Maternal diabetes mellitus
Fetal hydrops

*Urate = more specific Marker of PIH.*

Current literature favors the former view. Normal pregnancy is characterized by marked insensitivity to vasospastic influences. It may be that a loss of this insensitivity or the genesis of as yet unrecognized vasospastic agents underlies the net pressor state characteristic of PIH.

Edema indicates excess total ECF volume. The excess fluid is persistently misallocated to the extravascular compartment thus maintaining intravascular volume depletion. Secondary hyperaldosteronism plays a role in the maintenance of edema once it develops.

Depressed renal bloodflow (characteristic of all IVECF depleted states) may eventually lead to glomerular and tubular damage. Morphologic damage is preceded by functional aberration. IVECF depletion results in low renal tubular flow that promotes solute reabsorption. The solute best known to clinicians to behave in this manner is urea, however, urate is also increasingly reabsorbed and provides, for uncertain reasons, a more specific marker of PIH. (Note that the use of thiazide diuretics will falsely elevate uric acid levels.) Eventually significant proteinuria supervenes.

Eclamptic convulsions may be the result of focal cerebral hypoperfusion due to multiple small platelet thrombi or intense local vasospasm. Cerebral hemorrhage may also occur. Although convulsions become more likely as the blood pressure rises, eclampsia is not a manifestation of hypertensive encephalopathy.

*Clinical.* Determination of BP by the usual auscultatory methods is often the initial indicator of PIH. BP is typically labile and a reversal of the normal circadian rhythm for BP (resulting in higher readings during the nightime) may be observed. Edema is usually noted by the patient as an undue weight gain that is confirmed to be in excess of that expected for normal singleton pregnancy. The rate of weight gain is of greater importance than the magnitude of weight gain. Weight gain exceeding 1 kg/wk or 3 kg/month should prompt further investigation.

Proteinuria has been noted to vary in intensity from hour-to-hour thus perhaps implicating a functional rather than structural etiology. This variability may impair detection by random sample urinalysis. Proteinuria is usually the last component of the preeclamptic triad to appear, limiting its diagnostic worth.

*(handwritten margin notes:)*
① headache
② RUQ Pain
③ Oliguria  < 30 uc/hr
④ visual disturbances
⑤ hyperreflexia

Signs and symptoms associated with severe PIH and incipient convulsion include: (1) **headache,** usually frontal in location and resistant to nonsteroidal anti-inflammatory drug (NSAID) therapy; (2) **right upper quadrant or epigastric pain** due to subcapsular hepatic hemorrhage, with or without rupture of the capsule; (3) **oliguria** (< 400 ml/day or < 30 ml/hr); (4) **visual disturbances** including blurring, scintillations, or frank blindness (retinal arteriolar spasm or retinal edema, or both); and (5) **hyperreflexia.** The blindness associated with PIH is usually self-limited, resolving within several weeks of delivery once retinal edema resolves. Patients may also experience transient psychotic episodes that are amenable to neuroleptic therapy.

Although thrombocytopenia may be seen in milder forms of PIH, it is subclinical in all but the severely ill. Microangiopathic hemolysis, congestive heart failure, and liver failure are further indications of severe preeclampsia.

In addition to the serum urate level, other putative biochemical indices of PIH may include antithrombin-III and possibly serum $Fe^{++}$ and $Ca^{++}$ levels.

***Treatment.*** Close surveillance affords earlier detection, which has been shown to improve both maternal and fetal outcome. Termination of pregnancy leads to the resolution of PIH but the illness is frequently mild and the fetus immature so that temporization and induction of fetal pulmonary maturity with glucocorticoids is often attempted. This condition is managed in hospital with close monitoring of BP, daily weights, urinalysis, and daily inquiry as to the presence of the subjective manifestations of PIH. Bedrest and phenobarbital, 30 to 60 mg PO QID, for sedation may also be required.

**Thiazide diuretics are felt to be contraindicated** in PIH unless cardiogenic pulmonary edema supervenes because they (1) exacerbate the intravascular volume depletion, (2) invalidate plasma uric acid assays, and (3) often fail to relieve the hypertension of PIH. Diuretics may be used in patients with coincident hypertension that are refractory to antiadrenergics and vasodilators.

Further treatment will depend upon the severity of the illness, fetal maturity, and the condition of the cervix. Fetal well-being and maturity are assessed by biophysical parameters [nonstress test (NST) and/or contraction stress test (CST)], serial ultrasound (to determine fetal growth), and amniotic fluid L/S ratio determinations.

For patients with diastolic pressures up to 105 to 110 mmHg, antiadrenergic therapy (**methyldopa,** 0.5 to 3.0 g/day PO; **atenolol,** 50 to 100 mg/day PO; **propranolol,** 40 to 240 mg/day PO; **metoprolol,** 50 to 225 mg/day PO) is safe and usually adequate. Arteriolar vasodilators (**hydralazine,** 5 to 10 mg IV (IM) q20–30min; **diazoxide,** 30 mg IV boluses if hydralazine fails) are usually reserved for those with diastolic pressure > 110 mmHg. Diuretics are particularly hazardous (hypotension/shock) in cases of severe PIH.

In addition to the usual side effects associated with these medications it should be noted that methyldopa may be associated with neonatal tremors and beta-blockers can cause neonatal bradycardia and hypoglycemia. Preeclamptics are very sensitive to diazoxide, hence 30-mg aliquots are administered rather than the usual 300-mg dose. Diazoxide-induced hyperglycemia may preclude its use in mothers with diabetes mellitus. The following agents are contraindicated in pregnancy:

| Drug | Rationale |
| --- | --- |
| Nitroprusside | Fetal cyanide poisoning |
| Captopril | Fetal death in subhuman species |
| Ganglionic blockers (Trimethaphan) | Meconium ileus |

If conservative management fails to relieve the hypertension within 24 to 48 hours then induced labor is indicated. Other indications for induction of labor include: (1) declining renal function, (2) signs or symptoms of impending convulsion, (3) coagulopathy, and (4) fulminant liver failure. Delaying delivery in these situations benefits neither the mother nor the fetus. If the cervix is ripe once the patient has been stabilized, labor may be induced. If the cervix is firm and narrow, a cesarean section is indicated.

Although rapid fluid expansion is promulgated by certain researchers, this may exacerbate pulmonary or cerebral edema, or both. Nonetheless, it seems wise to be prepared to infuse colloid when administering vasodilators. Recall that the IVECF volume in PIH is depleted, therefore, isolated vasodilatation may result in precipitous hypotension and cardiovascular collapse. In addition the IVECF depletion is occasionally abruptly unmasked by delivery.

All evidence of preeclampsia usually resolves promptly after delivery but the mother warrants close attention for the first 24 hours because convulsions can occur for the first time during the puerperium (25% to 33%).

## Eclampsia

Defined earlier as the combination of preeclampsia and convulsions, eclampsia is classified as antepartum, intrapartum, or postpartum depending on the timing of the initial ictal event. Antepartum eclampsia can trigger the onset of labor. It is exceedingly rare for the convulsion to be the presenting complaint, almost always there is prodromal preeclampsia. As with generalized tonic–clonic seizures of other etiologies, the episode may be characterized by variable postictal somnolence. Seizures may recur during this period of somnolence. If death occurs, it results from cardiogenic pulmonary edema, intracerebral hemorrhage, or respiratory failure.

Laboratory parameters to be followed include complete blood count, platelet count, serum electrolytes (including $Mg^{++}$ and $Ca^{++}$), as well as liver and renal function tests.     *↳ urine $Ca^{2+}$ too*

*Treatment.* There exist several valid approaches to both BP and seizure control in PIH. Magnesium sulfate is commonly used as the anticonvulsant (in North America) and hydralazine as the antihypertensive agent (dosage given previously). The former agent may also possess a beneficial antihypertensive effect. Dosage regimen:     *＊ Mg for seizures + HTN*

- 20 ml of 20% magnesium sulfate IV stat (4 g)
- simultaneously 10 ml of 50% magnesium sulfate IM in each buttock*
- 10 ml of 50% magnesium sulfate IM q4h
*alternately a continuous iv magnesium infusion can be administered.

The patient is observed closely for evidence of hyporeflexia and declining respiratory rate, both suggestive of magnesium toxicity. Serum $Mg^{++}$ values should be measured:

| Normal | 0.65–1.15 mmol/L |
| Therapeutic range | ✳ 2.0–3.0 mmol/L |
| Toxic | > 5.0 mmol/L |

If respiratory depression is noted the magnesium infusion should be discontinued and calcium gluconate, 5 to 7 mg/kg by slow IV injection, may be considered. Alternate approaches for the treatment of eclamptic convulsions may use benzodiazepines, commonly diazepam. If continued seizure prophylaxis is required, longer-acting anticonvulsants (phenytoin, phenobarbital) should be commenced. Anticonvulsants should be continued through the first postpartum day.

## HEMOLYTIC DISEASE OF THE NEWBORN

Hemolysis as the result of isoimmunization (the development of antibodies to an antigen from a genetically dissimilar member of the same species) is a well-recognized phenomenon. Hemolytic disease of the newborn (HDNB) refers to a particular circumstance under which such isoimmunization occurs in one individual and subsequently causes clinically significant red blood cell (RBC) destruction in another individual (i.e., maternal isoimmunization with fetal anemia). Theoretically any antigen found on the fetal RBC that the mother does not possess can trigger an immune response in the mother. In point of fact the majority of offspring possess at least one antigen that they do not have in common with their mothers yet the incidence of HDNB is quite low.

The occurrence of clinical disease as a result of maternal isoimmunization to fetal RBC surface antigens is dependent on a number of factors including: (1) the existence of fetal RBC surface antigens the mother lacks, (2) the immunogenic capability of these antigens, (3) sufficient transplacental crossing of the antigen, (4) an adequate maternal immunologic response, and (5) the transfer of sufficient, "diffusable" (IgG) antibody back across the placenta to the fetus.

A large number of RBC surface antigens have been identified as causing HDNB but the vast majority of these antigens occur infrequently (e.g., Kell, Duffy, Kidd) in the population at large relative to the Rh group of antigens. The therapeutic introduction of anti-Rh$^+$(D) prophylaxis has resulted in these "rare" antigens being responsible for up to 50% of HDNB. The Rh and A/B/O antigen systems together account for the other half of HDNB.

## Rh Blood Group Incompatibility

Although there is no sex difference with respect to the incidence of the Rh$^+$(D) antigen (by far the most significant of the Rh group of antigens), there are definite racial differences. Asians have the highest incidence (~99%), followed by blacks (93%), and finally whites (87%). The incidence of Rh-induced HDNB can be expected to be highest in whites and lowest in Asians.

The pathophysiology of this disorder involves maternal exposure to the Rh$^+$(D) antigen (usually from the fetus), which induces a maternal immunoglobulin (IgG) response directed against this RBC surface antigen. Maternal IgG crosses the placenta into the fetal circulation where it induces hemolysis liberating excess hemoglobin for destruction (bilirubin). The presence of such antibodies in the fetal circulation is best determined by the direct antihuman globulin test (direct Coombs' test).

## Fetal Pathology

Generalized edema together with multiple body cavity effusions is referred to as **hydrops fetalis** and is the most severe manifestation of HDNB. This can sometimes be detected in utero by ultrasound as can the concomitant placental edema. Profound anemia stimulates marked extramedullary hematopoiesis (hepatosplenomegaly). Hepatic hematopoiesis overwhelms other liver functions with decreased coagulation factor synthesis (ecchymoses) and hypoalbuminemia, which promotes anasarca. Intra-abdominal organomegaly and ascites may lead to dystocia.

Hypoalbuminemia contributes to the misallocation of fluid to the EVECF space as does the "high cardiac output" heart failure due to severe anemia. The fetus may be grossly edematous, ecchymotic, limp, pallid, and dyspneic.

All hemolytic anemias, regardless of the etiology, produce an excess of lipid soluble bilirubuin-albumin (BA) or unconjugated bilirubin by overloading the normal metabolic pathways for the breakdown of heme pigments. Considerations unique to the fetal/neonatal age group arise due to the fact that the blood–brain barrier (BBB) is as yet poorly developed, thus permitting deposition of the excess pigment within the central nervous system (CNS), particularly the brainstem and the basal ganglia. This results in the clinical syndrome of **kernicterus (bilirubin encephalopathy)**. Clinically one observes spasticity of the extremities, head retraction, squinting, high-pitched cry, poor feeding, and convulsions. Residual evidence of the disease varies from sensorineural deafness to gross movement disorders and mental retardation. Note that the neonate may be asymptomatic initially and that not all of the above listed anomalies need be present to make the diagnosis. In utero the excess fetal BA crosses the placenta and is metabolized in the maternal liver. The absence of hyperbilirubinemia and its clinical correlates may thus persist for a variable length of time after delivery.

**Management.** The absence of the Rh⁺(D) antigen can be easily detected in the mother as can the occurrence of significant hemolysis in the fetus permitting more insightful therapeutic interventions. The degree of fetal hemolysis can be accurately quantitated by spectrophotometric analysis of the amniotic fluid. This information helps guide decisions regarding the appropriateness and timing of in utero **exchange transfusions** for the fetus.

The chief form of management is an attempt at primary prevention by means of passive immunization of the Rh negative [Rh⁻(d)] mother. All unsensitized Rh⁻(d) mothers with Rh⁺(D) partners should be given 1 ampule (300 mcg) of anti-Rh⁺(D) IM at 28 to 32 weeks' gestation to protect against active immunization resulting from "silent" fetal–maternal bleeds as well as for (1) spontaneous or induced abortions, (2) molar or ectopic pregnancy, and (3) amniocentesis. For clinically suspect fetal/maternal bleeds objective documentation can be achieved by the **acid elution test** performed on a sample of blood drawn from the mother. The fetal RBCs can be detected by virtue of the fact that they possess alkaline stable hemoglobin that stains more intensely by this method. Quantitation of the extent of the hemorrhage can be approximated by the following equation:

**(% Fetal RBCs per high power field) × Maternal hematocrit**

Dividing this value by 15 gives the number of 300-mcg ampules of anti-Rh⁺(D) that should be administered as it has been determined that 300 mcg of anti-Rh⁺(D) is sufficient to protect against a 15-ml bleed from the fetus to the mother. If the neonate is Rh positive [Rh⁺(D)], the mother should be given another ampule within 72 hours of delivery.

The anti-Rh⁺(D) that is administered interacts with the fetal RBCs encountered within the maternal circulation, thus preventing them from initiating an immune response that would sensitize the mother to form endogenous antibody to the Rh⁺(D) antigen. More importantly, the potential for an anamnestic response on subsequent challenge (next pregnancy with an Rh⁺(D) fetus) is thwarted. If given in the dosages suggested, there is only minimal transplacental passage of antibody and therefore no significant hemolysis. *RhoGAM induced hemolysis in fetus is minimal*

Rarely this schedule of prophylaxis fails because the mother was sensitized by prior transfusion or by maternal–fetal bleed while she herself was a fetus within an Rh⁺(D) mother. It is not practical to administer anti-Rh⁺(D) to all female Rh⁻(d) infants of Rh⁺(D) mothers. Whenever there is doubt as to whether the immune globulin should be administered or not, the general rule is that it should be given. The potential hazards to the fetus and subsequent fetuses of not administering the agent far outweigh the risks· of the relatively infrequent maternal side effects.

For those mothers that have been previously sensitized to Rh⁺(D), accurate knowledge of the gestational age of the fetus is prerequisite for the timing of any form of intervention. The degree of maternal sensitization is quantitated by assaying anti-Rh⁺(D) antibody titers in the maternal circulation. Titers of 1/16 or greater should prompt consideration of amniotic fluid bilirubin quantitation after 22 weeks LMP to plan further therapy. Amniotic fluid bilirubin concentrations correlate well with the degree of ongoing fetal hemolysis and as such are an indicator of the ''hostility'' of the intrauterine environment to the fetus.

Preterm delivery before 32 weeks LMP is contraindicated because of fetal immaturity and especially because infants with HDNB have a disproportionately increased incidence of respiratory distress syndrome (RDS) when compared with normal infants matched for gestational age. Thus, if indicated in utero fetal intraperitoneal exchange transfusion with Rh⁻(d) blood is performed in an attempt to preserve the relative safety of the intrauterine environment for the fetus until about 34 weeks LMP when the risks of repeat transfusion may exceed those of preterm delivery. Delivery can be accomplished by either oxytocin induction or cesarean section.

In utero fetal exchange transfusion is indicated if there is: (1) a prior history of Rh hemolytic disease; (2) high maternal anti-Rh⁺(D) antibody titer (titers drawn at ~22 weeks LMP); or (3) evidence of severe ongoing hemolysis in the fetus as ascertained by amniotic fluid bilirubin determinations. Note that the infused Rh⁻(d) RBCs are instilled in the fetal peritoneal cavity from which they are absorbed into the fetal circulation. Significant collections of ascitic fluid will impair transperitoneal RBC absorption. Whether to perform an immediate postpartum exchange transfusion for the neonate is determined by the hemoglobin and direct antihuman globulin test results on umbilical cord blood. Marked depression of the former and positivity of the latter are indications for exchange transfusion with fresh group O, Rh⁻(d) packed RBCs. If the anemia is not severe the requirement for transfusion is best determined by: (1) rate of rise of fetal bilirubin, (2) existence of other neonatal complications that make aggressive intervention undesirable, and (3) the degree of fetal maturity. Recall that other modalities are available for the treatment of rising neonatal bilirubin (if this is the only significant problem), e.g., ultraviolet light, barbiturates.

## Major A/B/O Blood Group Incompatability

Much remains to be explained about major A/B/O blood group incompatabilities and their relationship to hemolysis in utero or in the neonate. It is still uncertain how individuals acquire antibodies to the A/B/O system antigens they lack without proven exposure to them. The incidence of such incompatibilities (20%) far exceeds that of Rh group incompatibility yet the former causes clinically significant hemolysis in very few (5% of these cases, or 1% of all pregnancies). On closer inspection it becomes evident that the hemoglobin does fall and reticulocyte count and bilirubin concentration rise during the early neonatal period in cases of A/B/O mismatch. These subclinical alterations are much milder than those associated with Rh group incompatibilities.

To make the diagnosis of HDNB due to major A/B/O blood group

*[margin annotation: Ascites should be removed prior to Transfusion]*

*$I_g G$  Anti-A, Anti-B*

incompatability the following conditions must be met: (1) mother is type 0, (2) infant is type A, B, or AB, (3) neonatal jaundice commences within 24 hours of delivery, (4) fetal hemoglobin is down and reticulocyte count elevated, and (5) other blood group sensitizations have been ruled out. The postpartum management of these infants is similar to that for Rh-induced HDNB.

Notable distinctions from Rh-induced HDNB not already mentioned include: (1) the fact that direct antihuman globulin test results on cord blood are of no use in A/B/O blood group mismatch, (2) A/B/O blood group mismatch can, and frequently does, manifest in primigravidas due to preexisting sensitization, and (3) the incidence of stillbirth is not elevated in A/B/O-induced HDNB, thus operative preterm delivery is unwarranted. It has been noted that the existence of an A/B/O incompatability protects against the occurrence of Rh-induced HDNB.

## MEDICAL CONDITIONS IN PREGNANCY

This section deals with medical illnesses that are not unique to pregnancy but are sufficiently severe to potentially alter the outcome of pregnancy. Medical complications of pregnancy, PIH, and hemolytic disease of the newborn, are discussed in previous sections. Entities to be reviewed in this section include diabetes mellitus, cardiac disease, and pyelonephritis.

### Diabetes Mellitus

The prevalence of diabetes mellitus (DM) in pregnancy is 1 to 7 per 1000. Before the discovery of insulin it was highly unlikely that women with DM could successfully achieve pregnancy due to the severity of the metabolic aberration. Once pregnant, a 30% maternal and a 40% fetal mortality rate awaited. Better maternal plasma glucose control through the use of insulin has been credited with the marked improvement in maternal outcome and the (lesser) improvement in fetal outcome as well.

There exist two opposing influences on the plasma glucose concentration during pregnancy: (1) **those lowering maternal plasma glucose;** (a) the continual removal of glucose and amino acids from the maternal circulation into that of the fetus and (b) elevated basal levels of maternal insulin and increased insulin secretion in response to meals; (2) **those raising maternal plasma glucose;** (a) a rise in the antiinsulin hormone levels (cortisol, estrogen, progesterone, and placental lactogen) and (b) postreceptor insulin insensitivity in peripheral tissues. During the first 20 weeks of gestation the glucose lowering influences predominate with an overall decline in plasma glucose levels and, therefore, daily insulin requirements. During the latter half of pregnancy the antiinsulin hormone effect predominates increasing the daily insulin requirements.

Throughout pregnancy, however, the plasma glucose levels are prone to inordinate deviations in either direction. This "brittleness" is manifest as poor glucose tolerance postprandially and the ready appearance of ketosis during relatively short fasts.

*Diagnosis and Classification.* In the presence of typical symptomatology (polydypsia, polyuria, polyphagia, blurred vision, suboptimal weight gain early in pregnancy) a **fasting** venous plasma glucose (**VPG**), >7.8 mmol/L, or a **random VPG,** >11.1 mmol/L, is sufficient to diagnose diabetes mellitus. When the patient is asymptomatic, an **oral glucose tolerance test** (**OGTT**) is used to define both **DM** and **impaired glucose tolerance (IGT).** Indications for the OGTT include: (1) elevated fasting VPG on two occasions; (2) family history (first degree relatives) of DM; (3) prior macrosomic (>4.5 kg) infant; (4) prior fetal death or congenital anomaly; and (5) prior gestational diabetes mellitus.

The standardized test format calls for 3 days of unrestricted carbohydrate intake followed by a 10- to 14-hour (overnight) fast. The patient is then requested to rapidly ingest a 100-g glucose meal. Venous plasma glucose samples are then drawn at ingestion (time 0) as well as 1, 2, and 3 hours later

**TABLE 3-9. OGTT—DIAGNOSTIC CRITERIA**

|  | 0 hr | 1 hr | 2 hr | 3 hr |
|---|---|---|---|---|
| Within normal limits[a] (mmol/L) | <5.8 | <10.6 | <9.2 | <8.1 |

[a]National Diabetes Data Group, 1979.

(Table 3-9). The patient should remain seated and refrain from smoking during the entire test.

Gestational diabetes mellitus (GDM) is diagnosed if any two values exceed the limits of normalcy; gestational-impaired glucose tolerance (GIGT) is diagnosed if the 2-hour sample is 6.7 to 9.2 mmol/L. The qualifier "gestational" is added to indicate that the metabolic aberrations were initially detected during pregnancy. Patients with GIGT appear to be a heterogenous group with as yet no reliably predictable outcome. Patients with GDM have an increased risk of eventually becoming diabetic when not gravid (15% incidence over the subsequent 10 years).

The conventional classification of diabetes in pregnancy correlates reasonably with fetal outcome (Table 3-10).

*Management.* To detect subclinical GDM a screening test must be applied. Fasting VPG evaluations are inexpensive and rapid and the preferred screening test. By convention the fasting VPG assays are done at the initial visit and at ~28 weeks LMP. Urinary glucose concentrations are an index of plasma glucose concentrations provided the **glomerular filtration rate (GFR)** is constant. The ECF volume expansion of pregnancy greatly in-

**TABLE 3-10. CLASSIFICATION OF DM IN PREGNANCY IN THE WHITE POPULATION**

| Class | Age at Onset DM (yr) | Duration DM (yr) | Perinatal Mortality (%) |
|---|---|---|---|
| B | >20 | <10 | 7 |
| C | 10–20 | 10–19 | 9 |
| D | <10 | >20 | 15 |
| | **Special Classes** | | |
| A | GDM and GIGT | | 5 |
| F | Diabetic nephropathy (proteinuria or impaired creatinine clearance) before conception | | 30 ✻ |
| R | Proliferative diabetic retinopathy before conception | | 15 |
| H | Atherosclerotic heart disease before conception | | 25 |
| RF | Retinopathy and nephropathy | | 20 |

creases the GFR, rendering glucosuria fairly common and an unreliable index of plasma glucose homeostasis. OGTT is more expensive and time-consuming and should, therefore, only be performed when specific indications exist (usually at ~28 weeks LMP).

Patients with antecedent DM (classes B through RF) should be managed by a multidisciplinary team including an internist, neonatologist, and obstetrician. This approach should be extended to include patients who develop gestational diabetes mellitus. Primary care physicians should counsel sexually active female diabetics of childbearing age to present as soon as they desire to become, or are diagnosed, pregnant. Patients should be forewarned of the likelihood of several hospital admissions during their pregnancy (for optimization of plasma glucose control) so that they can organize their family and occupational responsibilities appropriately. Patients with retinopathy, nephropathy, or heart disease should also be informed of the potential long-term hazards to themselves and the high perinatal mortalities associated with these diabetic complications (Tables 3-11 and 3-12). Strict glucose control is imperative for optimal maternal and perinatal outcome and is highly patient dependent.

Patients who manifest GIGT should be followed with repeat fasting VPG evaluations at biweekly intervals and advised to maintain a 145-kJ/kg/day diet composed of 50% carbohydrate, 30% lipids, and 20% protein. The gestational age must be reliably determined (preferably sonographically) because it may alter delivery management. The patient should be seen biweekly until 32 weeks' gestation and weekly thereafter. At 32 weeks either weekly oxytocin challenge tests (OCTs) or biweekly NSTs are commenced. All patients should be carried to term if possible thus obviating routine amniocenteces for L/S ratio determination. Note that even

**TABLE 3-11. MATERNAL CONSEQUENCES OF DM IN PREGNANCY (0.5% MORTALITY)**

Worsened nephropathy (transient)
Worsened retinopathy
Accelerated coronary atherosclerosis
Increased incidence of operative delivery

**TABLE 3-12. FETAL CONSEQUENCES OF DM IN PREGNANCY (5–10% PERINATAL MORTALITY)**[a]

Macrosomia (class A–D)
Microsomia (class R, F, H, RF)
Seizure disorder/cerebral palsy (risk ↑ 5x)
Respiratory distress syndrome (30%)
Congenital malformation (15%)
Neonatal jaundice (30%)
Neonatal hypoglycemia (25%)
Neonatal hypocalcemia (20%)

[a]Neonatal and third trimester deaths are more frequent; spontaneous abortion rate is not increased by DM.

with an L/S ratio > 2.0, there is a 6% incidence of RDS in infants of diabetic mothers (IDM). If, however, **phosphatidyl glycerol** is also detectable in the amniotic fluid the risk of RDS falls to almost zero. Induced vaginal delivery is currently the favored method of delivery. Cesarean section is reserved for obstetric complications only. A fasting VPG should be performed 6 weeks postpartum to ensure that it has again returned to normal in GDM or GIGT patients.

## Cardiac Disease

Cardiac disease in pregnancy is composed of both congenital and acquired anomalies, in addition to surgically "corrected" heart disease. Although acquired cardiac disease (primarily acute and chronic rheumatic heart disease in this patient population) has declined over recent years, the number of women with surgically treated cardiac disease that survive beyond puberty has increased, thus the prevalence of cardiac disease in pregnancy remains 0.4% to 4.0%. Both maternal and fetal mortality are commonly reported in relation to the functional class (New York Heart Association) of the mother's cardiac disease (Table 3-13).

In addition to the physiologic alterations in the cardiovascular system (CVS) during pregnancy listed previously (increased heart rate, blood volume, preload and cardiac output; decreased total peripheral resistance), labor pain due to uterine contraction further stresses the system. Each uter-

TABLE 3-13. CARDIAC DISEASE IN PREGNANCY

| NYHA Class | Description | Maternal Mortality | Fetal Mortality |
|---|---|---|---|
| I | Symptomatic only with greater than ordinary activity | } 0.4% | Nil |
| II | Symptomatic during normal activity | | ~ |
| III | Symptomatic with minimal activity; asymptomatic at rest | } 7.0% | ~ |
| IV | Symptomatic at rest | | 30% |

NYHA, New York Heart Association. ~, data unavailable.

ine contraction is associated with a positive inotropic and chronotropic stimulus due to pain-induced adrenergic release and a 20% rise in venous return as the retracting uterus empties the contents of its vasculature into the systemic circulation. The puerperium is a period of variable CVS instability due to potentially rapid overcorrection of the ECF volume expansion of pregnancy by hemorrhage, diuresis, and lactation. The CVS generally returns to normal nonpregnant status within 1 to 2 weeks.

Complicating the diagnosis of cardiac disease in pregnancy are the many normal alterations of signs and symptoms (Tables 3-14 and 3-15). The chest x-ray (CXR) usually reveals upward and lateral displacement of the heart. The electrocardiagram (ECG) may exhibit left axis deviation and small Q waves in lead III. The diagnostic study of choice for the investigation of maternal cardiac disease in pregnancy is echocardiography with color Doppler. Right-heart catheterization without fluoroscopy can be accomplished without undue risk to the fetus and is often very helpful for managing acutely ill patients. Left-heart catherization is rarely required but can be performed with proper shielding for the fetus. Holter monitoring retains its usefulness in pregnancy for the detection of arrhythmias.

*General Management.* In general activity should be restricted and sudden or strenuous isometric exertion proscribed (Table 3-16). The patient should avoid exposure to temperature extremes and restrict sodium intake moderately. Factors that may exacerbate hyperdynamic circulation (anemia, hy-

**TABLE 3-14. COMMON CVS SIGNS AND SYMPTOMS DURING NORMAL PREGNANCY**

Dyspnea, fatigue; reduced exertional tolerance
Basilar pulmonary crackles
Waterhammer pulse
Nonsustained LV impulse   — 4th left IC space lateral to MCL
Nonsustained RV impulse   — LLSB
Nonsustained PA root      — 2nd left IC space
S1, increased intensity; prominent splitting
S2, expiratory splitting in the left lateral decubitus position
S3, common; may occasionally be followed by a short diastolic murmur due to after vibrations of the ventricular wall (apart from this, diastolic mumurs are uncommon in pregnancy)
S4, rare

**IC**, intercostal; **MCL**, midclavicular line; **LLSB**, lower left sternal border.

perthyroidism, hypertension, arrhythmia, infection/sepsis) must be treated aggressively to avoid precipitating acute pulmonary edema (15% maternal mortality). Individual judgment must be used with regard to the use of blood transfusions in the treatment of anemia. Pulmonary edema is treated in the same manner as for nonpregnant patients.

Although the American Heart Association does not recommend antimicrobial prophylaxis against bacterial endocarditis during delivery in patients with predisposing cardiac anomalies, most internists recommend it

**TABLE 3-15. MURMURS IN PREGNANCY**

| Benign Accentuated | Organic | |
|---|---|---|
| | *Attenuated* | *Accentuated* |
| Venous hum[a] | Mitral valve prolapse | Mitral stenosis |
| Pulmonic flow | Aortic regurgitation | Aortic stenosis |
| Brachiocephalic artery flow[a] | Mitral regurgitation | Pulmonic stenosis |
| Mammary souffle[b] | Hypertrophic cardiomyopathy | |

[a]Usually heard in the supraclavicular area; ablated by compressing the ipsilateral internal jugular vein.
[b]Systolic or continuous mumur bilaterally at second or third intercostal space; ablated by sitting up or pressure on or adjacent to the stethoscope.

**TABLE 3-16.** SPECIFIC CARDIAC DISORDERS IN PREGNANCY

| Disorder | Exacerbating Factors In Pregnancy | Specific Management |
|---|---|---|
| Mitral stenosis | ↑ CO and ↑ HR augment pressure gradient across mitral valve; ↑ LAP worsens pulmonary edema | Digoxin for AF; for positive past history of thromboembolism anticoagulate; 25% first diagnosed during pregnancy; closed valvotomy indicated for hemoptysis and intractable CHF |
| Aortic stenosis | ↓ TPR in face of fixed CO somewhat compensated by ↑ ECF volume of pregnancy but SHS causes sudden decompensation | Left lateral decubitus resting position advocated; avoid preload reduction (diuretics proscribed, generous fluid intake encouraged); vasodilators and negative chronotropic agents contraindicated |
| Cyanotic heart disease | All right-to-left shunts exacerbated by decline in systemic TPR | Rarely escapes surgery before pregnancy; high fetal morbidity and mortality; maternal mortality variable; treat as for aortic stenosis |
| Uncomplicated ASD, VSD, PDA | All left-to-right shunts are ameliorated by the decline in the TPR | None required |
| Mitral or aortic regurgitation | LV volume overloading lesions improved by low TPR, which facilitates forward flow of blood | None required |
| Hypertrophic cardiomyopathy and mitral valve prolapse | Forward flow ameliorated by ↓ TPR | None required |

*(handwritten in margin: supine hypotensive synd.)*

**AF,** atrial fibrillation; **ASD,** atrial septal defect (usually ostium secundum type); **CHF,** congestive heart failure; **CO,** cardiac output; **HR,** heart rate; **LAP,** left atrial pressure; **LV,** left ventricular; **PDA,** patent ductus arteriosus; **SHS,** supine hypotensive syndrome; **TPR,** total peripheral resistance; **VSD,** ventricular septal defect.

nonetheless. Common regimens include: penicillin, 2 million units IV or IM or ampicillin, 1.0 to 2.0 g IV or IM plus gentamicin, 1.5 mg/kg IM 30 minutes before delivery and twice more at 8-hour intervals. Substitute vancomycin (1.0 g IV over 1 hour) in penicillin-allergic patients.

Acute rheumatic fever is becoming increasingly rare during pregnancy due to several factors: (1) peak incidence occurs before puberty, (2) increased use of antibiotics for pharyngeal infections, and (3) advancing mean maternal age. Although the treatment is the same as for nonpregnant patients (bedrest and ASA) sudden death may complicate labor or the puerperium if there is ongoing active carditis.

**Cardiac disorders characterized by** <u>increased pulmonary vascular</u> **↑PVR** <u>resistance</u> (<u>Eisenmenger's syndrome</u>, primary pulmonary hypertension) have dismal prognoses in pregnancy (maternal mortality 30% to <u>70%</u> and 50%, respectively) and, therefore, pregnancy is contraindicated. If the patient is seen early in pregnancy, induced abortion may be suggested. If this not acceptable to the patient the treatment is similar to that for aortic stenosis (Table 3-16). <u>Marfan's syndrome</u> with significant aortic dilatation should be <u>handled in a similar manner because of the high risk of aortic dissection.</u> ✗

Vaginal delivery is currently the favored mode of delivery for mothers with cardiac disease. <u>Analgesia is beneficial but</u> <u>attention must be paid to the</u> <u>vasodilatory or negative inotropic effects</u>, or both, of some anesthetic agents, which may worsen outcome. *CABG*

Ischemic heart disease (<u>IHD</u>) is a relative rarity in pregnancy (1/10,000). Medical management is the same as for nonpregnant patients. Although coronary arterial bypass grafting (CABG) procedures have been successfully performed during pregnancy, a <u>unique and usually fatal</u> complication, <u>dissection of the left anterior descending artery</u>, has been noted ✗ during the puerperium.

Pregnancy is characterized by <u>relative supraventricular irritability</u>, thus increasing the incidence of <u>supraventricular tachyarrhythmias.</u> They generally respond well to <u>beta blockers, digoxin, or verapamil.</u> Cardioversion, if required, is <u>well tolerated by both mother and fetus.</u> Bradyarrhythmia is rare ✓ during pregnancy. The major harm of the supraventricular tachyarrhythmias is that they compromise diastolic filling time. Permanent pacemakers are well tolerated in pregnancy.

*Supraventricular Tachyarrhythmia*
*- respond to β blockers, dig, verapamil*
*- compromise diastolic Filling time.*
*- cardioversion well-Tolerated*

Surgical treatment of potential mothers with heart disease does not always lead to full correction of the problem, e.g., coarct repairs do not address the attendant risk of intracranial berry aneurysms or bicuspid aortic valves. Nonetheless, the major postoperative problem for the fetus is the attendant requirement for lifelong maternal anticoagulation. Warfarin is frankly teratogenic (epiphyseal abnormalities) and slow to reverse, thus heparin is favored during the first and third trimesters. Long-term heparin therapy throughout pregnancy, may lead to both fetal and maternal osteoporosis. Although glutaraldehyde-preserved porcine or bovine valves may reduce the requirement for anticoagulation, they experience accelerated rates of calcific degeneration in children and adults less than 30 years of age, therefore, mechanical valves are still preferable in this age group. Anticoagulation may also be necessary during pregnancy for intercurrent thromboembolic disease or refractory atrial fibrillation.

## Pyelonephritis    *more common on (R) side*

Pyelonephritis is inflammation of the renal pelvis and kidney due to bacterial infection. The patient usually presents with complaints consistent with lower genitourinary tract infection (dysuria, frequency and urgency) as well as fever and backache. The most common offenders are gram-negative enteric organisms, often *Escherichia coli*. Once bacterial cystitis occurs, upper genitourinary tract involvement is more likely in pregnancy due to progestin-induced dilatation of the renal drainage system, which facilitates upward spread of infection.

Agents useful in nonpregnant patients include tetracycline and sulfonamides in addition to nitrofurantoin, trimethoprim, co-trimoxazole, and ampicillin. **Tetracycline is teratogenic** and should thus be avoided during pregnancy. Sulfonamides (including that contained in co-trimoxazole) act to displace bilirubin from albumin, rendering the former available for CNS permeation and possible bilirubin encephalopathy (kernicterus). **Sulfonamide-containing agents should, therefore, be avoided during the last 2 weeks of gestation.**

**Asymptomatic bacteriuria** is defined as the presence of $> 10^8$ bacteria/L of urine in the absence of symptoms. The treatment of this condition in pregnant women has been shown to lower the incidence of acute pyelonephritis in the third trimester from 30% to 3%. Acceptable antibiotics include ampicillin, amoxicillin, or co-trimoxazole (as long as the above proviso is taken into consideration for the latter agent).

## EVALUATION OF FETAL WELL-BEING

Prenatal evaluation of the fetus presents the clinician with the unusual predicament of assessing a patient without the benefit of a physical examination. Several methods of obtaining useful information regarding fetal well-being are discussed here (Table 3-17).

### Maternal Estriols
In the past this was one of the cornerstones of prenatal fetal assessment. Normally there is a progressive rise in placental estriol synthesis throughout the course of pregnancy until just before term. A 50% decline or a 35% decline from the average of three prior values in maternal plasma estriol levels during pregnancy is a reliable indicator of impending fetal demise.

The disadvantages of maternal estriol determinations include (a) lack of etiologic information regarding fetal demise (b) high cost and (c) the prerequisites serial serum or 24 hr urine collection to derive useful information.

### Fetal Scalp Blood
Fetal scalp blood is reserved for the intrapartum period and is used to assess fetal acid/base status as an index of fetal distress. Both the $Pvco_2$ and the

**TABLE 3-17. METHODS TO EVALUATE FETAL WELL-BEING**

| Method | Noninvasive | Invasive |
|---|---|---|
| **Biochemical** | Maternal estriols | Fetal scalp blood analysis Amniocentesis |
| **Radiographic** | Ultrasound Plain radiography | |
| **Physical** | Nonstress test Fetal movements | Oxytocin contraction test |

$Pv_{O_2}$ are too evanescent to yield useful information. Of primary significance is the pH but one must recall that the samples are venous thus values as low as 7.20 are considered normal. The major disadvantage is the invasive nature of the procedure. There exists a possibility of fetal injury due to probe malplacement.

## Amniocentesis

Amniocentesis involves the withdrawal of amniotic fluid for analysis usually under sonographic control. Studies on the North American continent, both in the United States and Canada, have demonstrated a 1 per 200 postamniocentesis miscarriage rate above the expected fetal loss of 3.2%. All investigators currently agree that repeat aspirations, the use of needles larger than 20-gauge, and failure to locate the placenta sonographically are factors associated with increased complication rates.

Those complications reported include: (1) trauma to the fetus, placenta, umbilical cord, and maternal structures; (2) infection; and (3) preterm labor or induced abortion. Immediate examination of the fetus upon delivery for puncture sites may detect potentially lethal problems (thoracic puncture with pneumothorax). Fetal injury is more likely if there is a deficiency of fluid relative to fetal body size. Placenta is most optimally localized by sonography but in late pregnancy the suprapubic approach almost always obviates placental puncture. Immunologically significant fetal–maternal hemorrhage can occur even in the absence of placental damage, thus necessitating prophylactic passive immunization for all Rh-negative mothers having the procedure. Sonography before the procedure is required to establish placental location and the presence and location of adequate quantities of amniotic fluid for sampling.

Bloody taps, i.e., amniotic fluid contamination by either fetal or maternal blood significantly alters the interpretation of the results obtained. Fetal blood contamination leads to spuriously elevated alpha-fetoprotein levels if the hematocrit of the amniotic fluid is greater than 0.03 (3%). Maternal blood causes a dilutional depression of the lecithin/sphingomyelin (L/S) ratio falsely suggesting a greater degree of fetal immaturity.

Amniocentesis can be used for many different purposes depending on the information desired. Assays that may be performed include:

- Bilirubin concentration ΔOD 450
- Cytogenetic studies
- Fetal maturity indices
- Lecithin/sphingomyelin ratio (L/S ratio)
- Epithelial cell analysis

## Amniotic Bilirubin Concentration

The amniotic bilirubin concentration assay is used to detect the presence and severity of hemolytic disease of the newborn (HDNB). Normally the amniotic fluid bilirubin concentration falls during the latter half of pregnancy, but in the case of hemolytic disease the concentration is proportional to the degree of hemolysis. Even with clinically significant elevations routine biochemical assays are inadequate for bilirubin detection, thus continuous recording spectrophotometry is used. Operative preterm delivery may be warranted if amniotic bilirubin levels are very high.   ΔOD450

## Cytogenetic Studies

The intent of cytogenetic studies is to guide decisions regarding induced abortion. The amniocentesis is performed at about 15 to 17 weeks LMP. This assures the collection of sufficient quantities of fetal cells so that tissue culture results are available in time to induce a legal abortion. The major indication for such studies are advanced maternal age because of the associated rise in the number of chromosomal aberrations (trisomy 21 incidence increases from 1/250 at age 35 years to 1/40 at age 40 years). Karyotyping with fluorescent banding can detect a large number of such aneuploidies as well as balanced translocations that have been associated with congenital malformations. Biochemical assays to detect either abnormal elevations of the precursors of absent enzymes or of decreased enzyme activity itself in cultured fetal epithelial cells permits detection of inborn errors of metabolism.

## Fetal Maturity Indices

***Lecithin/Sphingomyelin Ratio.*** Functionally the fetal lungs do not mature  until the 35th to the 36th week LMP. Commencing at about the 20th week

35 - 36 wks LMP

LMP type II alveolar cells synthesize surfactants by a slow, inefficient methyl transferase pathway (major end product is phosphatidyl choline, lecithin). Surfactants are a collection of compounds that act to decrease surface tension in the sheet of fluid that overlays the alveolar epithelium. Surface tension is maximal at end expiration therefore surfactants act to prevent end-expiratory atelectasis. At 35 to 36 weeks LMP a more efficient phosphatidyl choline transferase pathway begins to predominate. Sphyngo-myelin, a nonsurface-active phospholipid, is produced at a constant rate throughout gestation, thus it can be used as a control value for comparison with lecithin production. Clinically this is assessed as the **lecithin/sphingo-myelin (L/S) ratio. When this ratio exceeds two (L/S > 2), at about the 35th week LMP, the lungs are functionally mature.** An L/S ratio of <2 is an index of fetal pulmonary immaturity and a high risk for RDS. RDS is relatively common despite L/S ratios >2 in patients that are infants of diabetic mothers or have HDNB.

*Epithelial Cell Analysis.* Staining the amniotic fluid with Nile blue sulfate reveals two types of cells, those that stain blue are epithelial in origin, whereas those that stain orange are of sebaceous gland origin. The detection of >10% to 20% orange cells is consistent with gestational age >36 weeks.

*Fetopelvic Ultrasound.* Although obstetric ultrasonography is discussed in depth in the next section, the sonographic biophysical profile of fetal well-being is outlined here. The sonographic portion of the profile assesses four parameters of fetal well-being: fetal breathing, fetal movements, fetal tone (limb or spine extension followed by flexion), and amniotic fluid volume. Each parameter is scored (0 if absent or insufficient, 2 if present or suffi-cient) for a possible total score of 8; if one of the parameters is absent a nonstress test is performed and also graded (0 to 2) for a possible total score of 10. A score of < 4 is suggestive of impending fetal demise, 4 to 6 is equivocal, and > 6 is normal.

  Plain radiography is limited to the diagnosis and management of abnor-mal fetal presentations in the late third trimester or intrapartum with breech presentation. Ultrasound has supplanted radiography because of the belief that high frequency pulsed sound is without significant side effects.

BPP
① Fetal breathing        ④ Amniotic Fluid Vol.
② Fetal movement
③ Fetal Tone

**TABLE 3-18. COMMON INDICATIONS FOR NST AND OCT**

Maternal diabetes mellitus
Pregnancy-induced hypertension
Chronic hypertension and pregnancy
?Intrauterine growth retardation
✓ Postterm gestation
Prior stillbirth
Meconium-stained amniotic fluid

*Physical Methods For Assessment of Fetal Well-Being.* One of the most informative parameters regarding fetal well-being is the response of FHR to hypoxic stress. The hypoxic stress can take the form of fetal movement (nonstress test, NST) or uterine contractions (contraction stress test, CST; also referred to as the oxytocin challenge test, OCT) (Tables 3-18 and 3-19). Uterine contractions can be induced by oxytocin infusion or may be spontaneous during normal labor.

The fetal CNS is very sensitive to hypoxic stress. The earliest discernable responses are certain reproducible FHR patterns. FHR pattern changes are clinically useful because they precede permanent hypoxic brain damage.

The fetal heart normally demonstrates **beat-to-beat variability.** Unlike adults, minor changes in sympathetic and parasympathetic tone in the fetus produce immediate changes in the FHR such that increased parasympathetic tone causes rapid, transient depression of the FHR followed by a rapid return to baseline, whereas increased sympathetic tone causes a rapid, transient elevation of FHR followed by return to baseline.

**TABLE 3-19. OCT CONTRAINDICATIONS[a]**

Prior classic cesarean section
Threatened preterm labor
Placenta previa
Premature rupture of the membranes
Abruptio placenta
Incompetent cervix
Multiple gestation

[a]NST is a benign procedure with no definite contraindications.

The modalities used to monitor fetal heart activity are direct (scalp electrode) or indirect (fetal ECG recordings taken over the maternal abdomen or sonographic detection of fetal cardiac valve activity). Scalp electrodes require breaching the integrity of the membranes, which invokes the risk of amnionitis if delivery is not relatively prompt. Transabdominal fetal ECG recordings are rarely satisfactory due to the electrical interference from maternal cardiac activity. Currently sonography of the fetal heart valves is the most popular noninvasive method for monitoring FHR patterns.

The monitoring of uterine activity is accomplished either by an open-ended intrauterine catheter or more commonly by external tocography. External tocography records **qualitative changes** in abdominal wall tension rather than giving quantitative values. Fetal movements can be monitored with the same instrument (as lesser variations in the tracing) or by having the mother employ a signal marker when movement is sensed.

*Procedure, Interpretation, and Intervention.* The NST and OCT are thought to be most reliable after 28 weeks LMP. The patient is placed in a semi-Fowler position (30 degree elevation of the head) while also laying on her left side (to obviate supine hypotensive syndrome). Recordings are made for a minimum of 20 minutes. For the NST, the initial absence of fetal movements is not abnormal (it is assumed that the fetus may be sleeping). Several maneuvers may be employed to stimulate him/her such as shaking the maternal abdomen or increasing maternal blood glucose level by having the mother eat. Before a tracing can be designated truly nonreactive, the FHR should be monitored for a full 40 minutes.

Unlike the NST, the OCT may induce labor and, therefore, should be performed with the delivery room facilities nearby. A continuous intravenous infusion of oxytocin is used starting with a dose of 0.5 mU/min and doubling it at 10-minute intervals until three regular contractions of 40- to 60-second duration occur within a 10-minute interval. The infusion is then discontinued and the mother and the fetus are monitored until uterine activity settles.

The **NST tracing** is interpreted as being reactive, nonreactive, sinusoidal, or unsatisfactory. A **reactive pattern** is characterized by: (1) beat-to-beat variability with the FHR changing by more than six beats per minute (bpm) occurring two to six times per minute; (2) at least three fetal movements accompanied by adequate increases in FHR during 20 minutes; and (3) an adequate increase in FHR consists of an increase of at least 15 bpm that is sustained for 15 to 20 seconds. A nonreactive pattern is characterized by: (1) beat-to-beat variability that does not fulfill the above criteria and (2) inadequate, occasional, or absent FHR response to fetal movement. A sinusoidal pattern, which is indicative of severe fetal distress, lacks any FHR increase in response to movement. The underlying tracing exhibits a 5- to 10-bpm amplitude and a 2- to 3-cycle per minute frequency. An unsatisfactory tracing is one in which the FHR is not detected.

The **OCT tracing** is interpreted as being positive, negative, hyperstimulation, or unsatisfactory. A positive tracing (late decelerations) is associated with fetal distress due to uteroplacental insufficiency. This pattern is defined as consisting of persistent late decelerations of the FHR. Specifically there is a 20- to 30-second delay after the onset of uterine contraction before the FHR begins to decelerate; the FHR nadir occurs after uterine contraction intensity peaks and recovery toward baseline FHR begins to occur after uterine contraction is complete. This pattern becomes even more ominous if normal beat-to-beat variability is lacking between contractions. A **negative** tracing (early decelerations) suggests no fetal distress. In such tracings the decline in the FHR and rise in uterine tone are simultaneous, as are the FHR nadir and uterine tone peak as are their return to their respective baseline values. (**Variable** decelerations are characterized by variability in both the temporal relationship between FHR and uterine tone and in the morphology of the FHR waveforms themselves. They are associated with fetal distress due to umbilical cord compression.)

The remaining two interpretations refer to technical aspects of the test. **Hyperstimulation,** as the name implies, refers to excessive uterine activity specifically, contractions occurring more frequently than every 2 minutes and lasting longer than 90 seconds. An **unsatisfactory** OCT tracing is one in which less than three contractions occur within a 10-minute interval or the quality of the tracing is poor.

Possible interventions based on the findings of these tests are shown in Figure 3-1.

Optimal management involves complimentary use of the biophysical

NST high False ⊕ rate of 25-33%

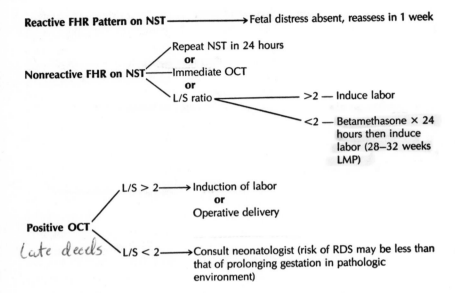

Reactive FHR Pattern on NST ────────→ Fetal distress absent, reassess in 1 week

Nonreactive FHR on NST
  ╱ Repeat NST in 24 hours
     **or**
  ── Immediate OCT
     **or**
  ╲ L/S ratio ──── >2 — Induce labor
                    <2 — Betamethasone × 24 hours then induce labor (28–32 weeks LMP)

Positive OCT
  ╱ L/S > 2 ──→ Induction of labor
               **or**
               Operative delivery
  ╲ L/S < 2 ──→ Consult neonatologist (risk of RDS may be less than that of prolonging gestation in pathologic environment)

*Late decels*

**Figure 3-1.** Possible interventions based on NST or OCT findings.

profile, NST, and OCT. The former is benign and can thus be used as a screening test for pregnancies thought to be at high risk of fetal/neonatal loss. The NST has a relatively high false-positive rate (nonreactive pattern in 25% to 33%). The OCT is a more specific test but runs the risk of preterm labor.

## ULTRASOUND

Ultrasound has supplanted standard radiography as the imaging procedure of choice during pregnancy because it lacks any serious side effects and provides reasonable resolution.

Pelvic sonography requires a full bladder to provide an "ultrasonic window" through which the sound waves can pass unimpeded. Real time

*[handwritten top margin:]* Assess Fetal age { CRL — 1st Trimester / BPD > 13, 14 wks

scanning equipment can accurately delineate fetal presentation and placental location as well as provide more credible evidence of fetal demise than routine radiography. Unfortunately the round ligament, the ovarian ligament, the fallopian tubes, and the ovaries cannot be distinguished as separate entities so they are referred to generically as the adnexae. Intrauterine devices can be easily located with ultrasound. The following fetal structures are predictably detectable:

| | |
|---|---|
| Gestational sac | 5 wk LMP |
| Fetal echoes | 6 wk LMP |
| Fetal cardiac activity | 7–8 wk LMP |
| Placenta | 10 wk LMP |
| Fetal skull | 12 wk LMP |

**Fetal gestational age** can be estimated as early as the first trimester by measurements of the longest dimension of echoes available, the crown–rump length (CRL). Accurate assessments of fetal age can be made after 13 to 14 weeks LMP based on the biparietal diameter (BPD).

The normal fetal gestational sac is characterized by: (1) oval shape, (2) complete margin, and (3) well-delineated echoes. Deviation from this appearance is presumptive evidence of **fetal demise.** A double outline of the fetal head ("halo") and body is consistent with Rh isoimmunization (fetal edema), diabetes mellitus, or fetal demise from other cause. Further ultrasound findings consistent with fetal demise include: (1) poorly defined falx cerebri, (2) abnormal head shape, (3) absence of fetal motion during the study, (4) failure of BPD to increase on serial scans, and (5) failure, on real time equipment, to visualize cardiac activity after seventh week. *[handwritten margin: halo]*

Assessment of the **placenta** by ultrasound permits **localization** for amniocentesis, to rule out placenta previa or to follow a low-lying placenta. The placenta normally appears to migrate cephalad due to disproportionate growth of the lower uterine segment. Calcification of the intercotyledonary septa is normal after 36 weeks LMP but if seen before 32 weeks LMP it suggests premature placental senescence (intrauterine growth retardation, maternal hypertension, uteroplacental insufficiency). **Intrauterine growth retardation (IUGR)** may be suggested by serial ultrasounds showing poor fetal growth.

*[handwritten bottom margin:]*
Calcif of septa @ 36 LMP NL
If seen before 32 wks suggests premature placental aging.

*Dystocia = abnl Labor*

**TABLE 3-20. OBSTETRIC APPLICATIONS FOR SONOGRAPHY**

Early confirmation of pregnancy
Identifying fetal number, anomalies, death
Estimating fetal age
Placental localization
Identifying placental anomalies (senescence,
  molar pregnancy)
Amniotic fluid volume assessment

---

A uterus larger than expected for dates can be the result of incorrect dates, multiple pregnancy, polyhydramnios or molar pregnancy. Multiple pregnancy is suggested by the presence of multiple gestational sacs with a fine septae separating them. **Polyhydramnios** can be directly visualized and should suggest the possibility of neural tube defect (associated with elevated serum alpha-fetoprotein) or discontinuity of the gastrointestinal tract (associated with trisomy 21). The combination of bilateral ovarian cysts (theca lutein cysts), markedly elevated maternal serum human chorionic gonadotropin (HCG) levels, and a highly echogenic intrauterine pattern with a "snowstorm" appearance is highly suggestive of molar pregnancy.

*α-FP*
*mole*

## DYSTOCIA

Dystocia is defined as abnormal labor. Labor can be rendered abnormal by: (1) inadequate myometrial contractions (first stage of labor); (2) inadequate voluntary muscle contraction (second stage of labor); (3) fetal malpresentation or malformation; and (4) an abnormal birth canal. The latter two factors are considered together as fetopelvic disproportion (FPD) or cephalopelvic disproportion (CPD).

*CPD*

The first stage of labor has been arbitrarily divided into two phases, latent and active. During the **latent phase** the cervix softens and the cervical canal is ablated as the lower uterine segment forms. These events are for the most part clinically inapparent, hence aberrancies are often diagnosed retrospectively. During the **active phase** the external cervical os dilates. Abnor-

*Latent phase = cx softens, cx canal ablated,*
*Active phase = os dilates*

malities of the active phase are detected by repeat pelvic examination (Table 3-21).

Friedman curves are a way of depicting the relationship between cervical dilatation and time, thus a normal curve is relatively flat (slope <1) during the latent phase and then steep (slope >1) during the active phase. The slopes of these phases differ for primigravid and multiparous women (Figure 3-2).

There are two clinically distinguishable forms of uterine insufficiency. Hypotonic uterine insufficiency is characterized by low basal myometrial tone with preservation of the normal cornual–cervical progression of myometrial contraction. The uterus is easily indented (through the abdominal wall) during peak contraction and contractions generally weaken and cease. This form of uterine insufficiency usually underlies secondary arrest of dilatation (i.e., occurs after active phase has commenced). Oxytocin may successfully augment uterine activity but is only indicated if the existence of CPD has been ruled out.

Hypertonic (or incoordinate) uterine insufficiency is characterized by normal or elevated basal myometrial tone but the cornual–cervical progression of uterine contraction is disrupted. The patient experiences disproportionate pain for the degree of fetal descent or cervical dilatation, or both. This form of uterine insufficiency is often responsible for prolongation of the latent phase. Oxytocin use may exacerbate the discomfort.

During the second stage of labor the mother usually experiences an overwhelming urge to bear down or push. Inadequacy of voluntary muscle

**TABLE 3-21. DYSTOCIA DUE TO UTERINE INSUFFICIENCY**

| Diagnosis | Definition | | Management |
| | Primigravidas | Multiparas | |
|---|---|---|---|
| Prolonged latent phase | > 20 hr | > 14 hr | Therapeutic rest |
| Protracted active phase | < 1.2 cm/hr | < 1.5 cm/hr | Observe |
| Secondary-arrest of dilatation | > 2 hr | > 2 hr | Minimal CPD, trial labor; Marked CPD, cesarean section |

CPD, cephalopelvic disproportion.

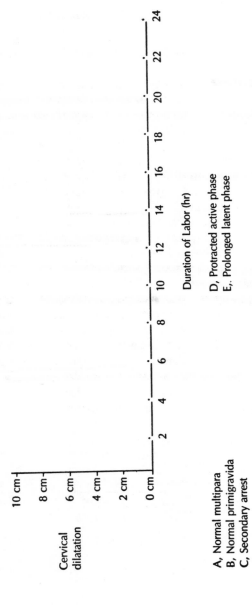

Cervical
dilatation

10 cm
8 cm
6 cm
4 cm
2 cm
0 cm

2  4  6  8  10  12  14  16  18  20  22  24

Duration of Labor (hr)

A, Normal multipara
B, Normal primigravida
C, Secondary arrest

D, Protracted active phase
E,. Prolonged latent phase

**Figure 3-2.** Sample Friedman curves.

CPD

contraction during the second stage is frequently the result of excessive anesthesia or sedation. Other causes include an emotionally immature or ill-prepared mother or neuromuscular disorders causing paralysis. This problem is best treated by prevention which includes adequate preparation of the patient for labor.

**Cephalopelvic disproportion** refers to the inability of a given fetus to pass through a given pelvis. Factors predisposing to CPD may include:

| **Maternal** | **Fetal** |
|---|---|
| Contracted pelvis | Macrosomia (>4.5 kg) |
| Pendulous abdomen | Anomalous body |
| Pelvic mass lesion | (e.g., hydrocephalus) |
| (fibroid, full bladder, cyst) | Deflection attitudes |
| Congenital uterine anomaly | Multiple pregnancy |
| | Placental anomalies (size, shape) |

Significant historical features in the diagnosis of dystocia include details of prior births (number and condition of children at birth, duration of prior labors, and method of delivery). A family history of prolonged labors, prolonged involuntary infertility, and maternal age >35 years are associated with a higher incidence of dystocia in primigravidas. Maternal abdominal examination should permit diagnosis of fetal position, presentation, and attitude but may also provide evidence of abdominopelvic mass lesions (e.g., full bladder or rectum), gross fetal anomaly, or polyhydramnios. Pelvic examination should provide at least a gross assessment of the adequacy of the birth canal (e.g., diagonal conjugate, pelvic sidewalls, and sacral prominence, subpubic angle).

The terminology applied to the diagnosis of fetopelvic relations is as follows:

- *Lie:* The relationship between the long axis of the fetus to that of the mother. In simpler terms the lie describes the relationship of fetal to maternal spine.
- *Presentation:* The fetal part that overlies the pelvic inlet at the beginning of labor, e.g., cephalic (head), breech (buttocks), or shoulder.
- *Presenting Part:* The most dependent fetal part nearest the cervix.

- *Attitude:* The relationship between the fetal parts themselves; **flexion** for chin to chest and **extension** for occiput apposed to the back.
- *Denominator:* An arbitrarily chosen reference point located on the presenting part of the fetus, e.g., occiput, mentum, frontum, sacrum.
- *Position:* The relationship of the denominator to the maternal pelvis. There are eight positions spaced equally every 45 degrees around a full 360-degree circle.

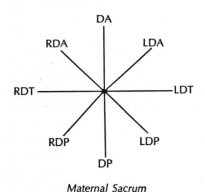

*Maternal Symphysis*

*Maternal Sacrum*

**L,** Left (of maternal pelvis)
**R,** Right (of maternal pelvis)
**D,** Denominator
**A,** Anterior
**T,** Transverse
**P,** Posterior
**e.g., LOA,** left occiput anterior

## Consequences of Dystocia

The effects of dystocia are borne by the process of labor and the two participants in the process, namely the mother and the fetus.

With respect to labor there is (1) decreased efficiency of uterine contractions with prolongation of labor; (2) slower cervical dilatation promoting the formation of pathologic retraction rings (associated with uterine rupture); (3) increased incidence of premature spontaneous rupture of membranes (SROM); and (4) failure to progress with the fetal presenting part remaining high.

Maternal exhaustion is more common with prolonged labor of any cause. In addition there is an increased risk of peripartum uterine hemorrhage because of the greater chance of trauma and uterine atony. Chorioamnionitis due to premature rupture of the membranes (PROM) and puerperal endometritis are also more common.

Neonatal consequences are primarily due to prolonged labor: (1) excessive molding, (2) greater risk of hypoxic/ischemic insult, (3) intrauterine death, and (4) umbilical cord prolapse.

*Management.* The management of CPD includes cesarean section whenever a marked degree of disproportion exists and forceps delivery when minor CPD is suspect and only rotation or flexion are required to permit vaginal delivery. Symphysiotomy (transection of the symphysis pubis) is another less favored technique for facilitating vaginal deliveries in patients with CPD.

In situations where the degree of CPD is thought to be borderline a trial of labor is permissible because adequate uterine activity may be capable of overcoming minor CPD with a good fetal and maternal result. Active labor should be allowed to commence spontaneously but it may be enhanced thereafter by amniotomy or uterotonic agents.

## PROLAPSE OF THE UMBILICAL CORD

Defined as the umbilical cord being below or beside the presenting part of the fetus, this condition occurs in less than 1% of pregnancies. The significance of the condition derives from the disproportionately high fetal mortality rate (35%) if the diagnosis is delayed. Labor is unaffected by the prolapsing cord and the mother is only at risk of harm due to overzealous attempts at vaginal delivery. Five factors increase the risk of umbilical cord prolapse during labor: (1) failed engagement, (2) small or anomalous fetus, (3) polyhydramnios (flushing effect of excess fluid), (4) rupture of the amniotic membranes before engagement of the presenting part (iatrogenic or spontaneous), and (5) fetal malpresentation (e.g., breech).

The prolapsed cord may be visible beyond the introitus or the diagnosis may be made during pelvic examination or by FHR recordings (**variable**

**decelerations).** Once diagnosed, gentle pressure should be applied to the presenting part and the mother placed in either the knee–chest or the Trendelenburg position to relieve umbilical cord compression. Oxygen is provided to the mother by mask and the fetal heart rate monitored frequently. Further measures are dependent on the clinical situation. If the cervix is fully dilated, the presentation cephalic, and the head low down, forceps delivery is attempted. In all other situations (excluding fetal death or anomaly where no intervention is warranted), cesarean section is indicated. Manual attempts at cervical dilatation by force or incision are unjustifiable.

## PRETERM LABOR

Preterm labor is defined as the onset of regular uterine contractions with cervical dilatation, effacement, and fetal descent before 37 weeks LMP. Although the incidence is only about 7%, preterm labor is the most common cause of perinatal morbidity and mortality. Some terminology warrants review at this point:

- *Term Labor:* Onsets after 37 weeks but before 42 weeks LMP.
- *Postterm Labor:* Onsets after 42 weeks LMP.
- *Low Birth Weight:* Fetal weight <2500 g regardless of gestational age.
- *Small for Gestational Age (SGA):* Variably defined as birthweight < the 10th percentile for gestational age or birthweight < 2 standard deviations below the mean (the third percentile) for gestational age. (Synonymous with small-for-dates, whereas IUGR refers to the process that results in SGA).
- *Large for Gestational Age (LGA):* Similarly defined as either birthweight > than the 90th percentile for gestational age or birthweight > 2 standard deviations above the mean (the 97th percentile) for gestational age.

Accurate diagnosis is important if unnecessary and possibly harmful interventions are to be avoided. Preterm labor should only be diagnosed when the following criteria are met: (1) cervix 2 cm dilated or at least 75%

effaced and (2) progressive dilatation or effacement of the cervix occurs during the period of observation.

Preterm delivery may be initiated intentionally by the obstetrician in the management of disorders that render the uterus "hostile" to the fetus, e.g., PIH, maternal DM, hemolytic disease of the newborn. Two common causes of preterm labor not discussed elsewhere are cervical incompetence and premature rupture of the membranes (PROM). They will be discussed in this section.

Preterm infants with birthweight between 700 and 1500 g have a 50% survival rate. Preterm neonates are much more sensitive to general anesthetics and narcotic analgesics. Such agents should be avoided and continuous FHR monitoring should be used. Preterm infants can sustain serious injury (e.g., intracranial hemorrhage) despite minimal obstetric trauma. Precipitate delivery is avoided specifically by (1) avoiding amniotomy, (2) performing episiotomy, or (3) delivery by low forceps to dilate the perineal portion of the birth canal.

**Management.** The most satisfactory form of management for preterm labor is its prevention by proper management of maternal and fetoplacental conditions listed in Table 3-22. Failing this, the goal becomes the prolongation of labor as long as medically advisable. This is accomplished primarily by tocolytic medications.

**TABLE 3-22. ETIOLOGY OF PRETERM LABOR**

| Fetoplacental | Maternal |
|---|---|
| Premature rupture of membranes | Cervical incompetence |
| Placental insufficiency (PIH, maternal DM) | Uterine anomaly (myoma, synechiae, congenital malformation) |
| Uterine distension (polyhydramnios, macrosomia, multiple pregnancy) | Serious maternal illness (e.g., pyelonephritis) |
| Late vaginal hemorrhage[a] | Trauma |

[a]Third trimester hemorrhage; Extravasated blood renders myometrium irritable (i.e., more responsive to contractile stimuli).
**DM,** diabetes mellitus; **PIH,** pregnancy-induced hypertension.

## Respiratory Distress Syndrome
**RDS is the most common cause of morbidity and mortality for preterm infants.**
Prematurity is the single most common factor associated with infant death and 45% of deaths in the neonatal period (the first 7 days of postnatal life) are attributable to RDS. Preterm infants also have 12 times the risk of perinatal hypoxia and 5 times the risk of intracranial hemorrhage when compared with infants delivered at term. Functionally the fetal lungs do not mature until the 35th to the 36th week LMP. Commencing at about the 20th week LMP type II alveolar cells synthesize surfactants by a slow, inefficient methyl transferase pathway (major end product is phosphatidyl choline, lecithin). Surfactants are a collection of compounds that act to decrease surface tension in the sheet of fluid that overlays the alveolar epithelium. Surface tension is maximal at end expiration therefore surfactants prevent end-expiratory atelectasis. At week 35 to 36 LMP a more efficient (phosphatidyl choline transferase) pathway is activated. Sphingomyelin, a nonsurface-active phospholipid, is produced at a constant rate throughout gestation, and is used as a control value to which lecithin production is compared. Clinically this is assessed as the lecithin/sphingomyelin ratio. When this ratio exceeds two (L/S > 2) at about the 35th week LMP, the lungs are functionally mature.

It had been noticed that intrauterine stress of diverse cause was associated with increased endogenous release of fetal glucocorticoids and a lower than usual incidence of RDS. As a result it was suggested that the administration of exogenous steroids would be equally effective in non-stressed fetuses delivering preterm. This remains controversial and some authorities remain unconvinced of its salutary effects. If the fetus is between 28 and 32 weeks LMP and the L/S ratio < 2, one should attempt to delay delivery by 24 hours and consider the administration of betamethasone 12 IM q12h to the mother.

Contraindications to glucocorticoids include: (1) sufficient endogenous stress (PIH, maternal DM); (2) fetomaternal infection (defenses are further compromised by steroids); and (3) uteroplacental insufficiency (a contraindication to prolonging labor in any situation).

Side effects include reports of an increased incidence of neurologic deficit with or without intracranial hemorrhage. In some animal species glucocorticoids have been found to hasten labor. Finally, the mortality of PIH may be worsened

# Tocolytics

Tocolytics are drugs that inhibit labor. Their efficacy is equivocal. They are said to be effective only during the latent phase of the first stage of labor. ✗ Once the active phase commences with rapid cervical dilatation, especially if SROM has occurred, cessation of labor is highly unlikely.

There are three classes of agents: (1) beta adrenergic agonists (isoxuprine, ritodrine, salbutamol); (2) prostaglandin synthetase inhibitors (indomethacin, ASA); and (3) others (alcohol, $MgSO_4$). The beta agonists stimulate uterine $beta_2$ receptors leading to uterine relaxation. The prostaglandin inhibitors prevent synthesis of the principle uterotonic prostaglandin $PF_{2\alpha}$. Other agents act by poorly understood mechanisms.

*$\beta_2$ receptors        $PF_{2\alpha}$*

## TABLE 3-23. TOCOLYTIC MEDICATIONS

| Agent | Dosage Regimen | Adverse Reactions |
|---|---|---|
| Isoxuprine | 80 mg in 500 ml 5%D/W IV @ 30 ml/hr to max 120 ml/hr until 24 hr after contractions cease, then 30–80 mg PO q3h | *Maternal:* vasodilatation with hypotension and tachycardia; myocardial ischemia; *Fetal:* neonatal hypoglycemia |
| Ritodrine | 150 mg in 500 ml 5%D/W IV @ 20 ml/hr; increase by 10 ml/hr q15min to max 120 ml/hr (100 mcg/min to 600 mcg/min) for 12 hr after contractions cease; 30 min before IV stops, start 10 mg PO q2h × 24h then 10–20 mg PO q4–6h | Same as above but less hypotension |
| Salbutomol* *Albuterol* | 5 mg in 500 ml 5% D/W IV @ 60 ml/hr; increase by 30 ml/hr q10min to max 120 ml/hr for 6 hr after contractions cease; 4 mg PO q6h × 48h | Same as isoxuprine |
| Indomethacin | 100 mg PO BID or 25 mg PO q6h and 100 mg PR QHS | May promote premature closure of ductus arteriosus; few if any maternal side effects |

*Albuterol in USA.

*Cervical incompetence= recurrent mid Trimester sp Ab*
*c̄ painless cervical dilatation*
  *1. idiopathic*

**94**     **OB/GYN NOTES**     *2. excessive D+C*
  *3. Prior cone*

Indications and contraindications are discussed for the entire group, while selected agents are described in tabular form (Table 3-23). To initiate tocolytic therapy one must satisfy the following criteria: (1) the fetus and the uteroplacental environment must be healthy; (2) labor must still be in its earliest stages (cervical dilatation < 5 cm and no SROM); (3) the degree of prematurity should be sufficient to warrant intervention (estimated birthweight < 2500 g or gestational age < 35 weeks LMP); and (4) there must be no contraindication to prolonging labor.

Contraindications to tocolytics include: (1) fetus is unhealthy (IUGR, severe malformation, dead); (2) hostile uteroplacental environment (PIH, maternal DM, hemolytic disease of the newborn, amnionitis); (3) incipient active phase of labor (SROM, bulging membranes); or (4) maternal hemodynamic instability, which may be exacerbated by beta agonist agents.

## Cervical Incompetence

The clinical syndrome of recurrent midtrimester spontaneous abortions with painless cervical dilatation is described as cervical incompetence. Etiologies may include excessive dilatation during dilatation and curettage (D & C) and prior cone biopsy of the cervix. The majority of cases are idiopathic. The presentation is typically midtrimester with a dilated, effaced cervix, the membranes either having ruptured or still bulging.

The diagnosis can also be made while nonpregnant if a #8 Hegar dilator can be passed easily through the cervical canal, a Foley catheter with 1 ml of fluid in the balloon can be easily withdrawn from the uterus, or a hysterosalpingogram demonstrates an internal os > 8 mm.

**TABLE 3-24. INDICATIONS, CONTRAINDICATIONS AND COMPLICATIONS OF CERVICAL CERCLAGE**

| Indications | Contraindications | Complications |
|---|---|---|
| Precipitate and painless labor | Amnionitis | Suture tears |
| Cervical os >2 cm at midtrimester | SROM | Infection |
| Prior midtrimester spontaneous abortion | True labor ongoing | Inadvertent amniotomy |
| Prior cerclage | Vaginal hemorrhage | Preterm labor |

*PROM*

*14-16 wks LMP*

The therapeutic approach consists of tracheloplasty if nonpregnant or cervical cerclage by the method of either Shirodkar or Macdonald. This is usually performed early in the second trimester (14 to 16 weeks LMP) with removal of the stitches ~2 to 3 weeks before term.

## Premature Rupture of the Membranes

Premature rupture of the membranes (PROM) is defined as rupture of the membranes more than 1 hour before the onset of labor. Frequently (~70%) labor commences within the subsequent 48 hours. The duration of this period of latency is usually inversely related to gestational age and fetal weight.

Premature rupture of the membranes increases the risk of chorioamnionitis, but this can usually be treated successfully with prompt delivery and antibiotics. Fetal hazards of PROM include: (1) with subsequent fetal/neonatal infection (often pneumonia) and (2) preterm labor (20% of PROM) with its increased likelihood of malpresentation (usually breech) and therefore cord prolapse (the presenting part fits the maternal pelvis less snugly).

*Management (Fig. 3-3).* PROM must be documented objectively (see section on labor). Digital pelvic examination should be avoided and only sterile speculum examination performed (to document PROM and for taking cervical smears for culture and sensitivity [C/S]). FHR should be monitored throughout labor.

Conservative management usually consists of hospital admission for close observation (daily temperature, twice weekly cervical swabs for C/S, daily white blood cell count) and bedrest. NSTs and ultrasounds are performed once or twice each week. Any evidence of amnionitis warrants induction of labor. Very occasionally conservative management can be done on an outpatient basis provided vital signs are stable and vaginal fluid loss is not excessive. Coitus, douches, and tampons are proscribed. The patient must take her temperature reliably on a TID schedule. Should fever occur, hospital admission and induction are indicated.

Upon delivery the neonate should have the following sites cultured; nose, throat, external auditory meatus, gastric aspirate, blood, cerebrospinal fluid, and urine in addition to a complete blood count and differential count

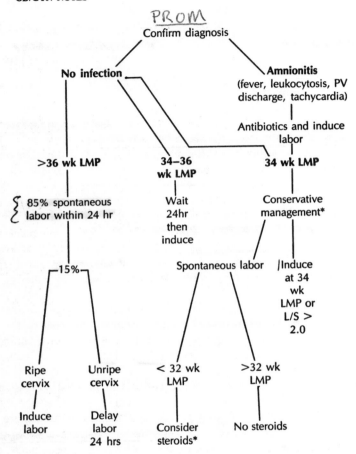

*Steroids may be given before the onset of spontaneous labor as part of the conservative management of this group.

**Figure 3-3.** Management profile for premature rupture of the membranes.

*Hellin's Law*

and chest x-ray. Antibiotics should be commenced empirically for both the infant and the mother.

## MULTIPLE PREGNANCY

Multiple pregnancy refers to the presence of more than one fetus during a single gestation, whether they are anatomically separate or not. Hellin's law estimates the incidence of multiple pregnancy by the following equation:

$$r = (1/89)^{n-1},$$

where $r$ = incidence and $n$ = the number of fetuses.

Thus the incidence of twins is 1/89, whereas that of triplets is ~1/8100. The total number of fetuses developing during a single pregnancy is inversely related to individual fetal birthweight and duration of pregnancy.

| # of Fetuses | Mean Birthweight | Duration of Gestation |
|---|---|---|
| 1 | 3.4 kg | 40 wk LMP |
| 2 | 2.4 kg | 37 wk LMP |
| 3 | 1.8 kg | 35 wk LMP |

In general singletons carried for the same length of gestation are 200 to 800 g heavier at birth.

*Physiology and Etiology.* A zygote is defined as the cell that results from the union of sperm and ovum until it undergoes its first division. Multiple pregnancies are referred to as either **monozygotic** or **polyzygotic.** The former are derived from a single fertilized ovum that experiences complete cleavage of the blastoderm. Partial cleavage results in conjoined twins. Polyzygotic fetuses are each derived from a separate zygote and thus possess differing genotypes (nonidentical sibs).

The cause of multiple pregnancy is unknown but an increased incidence of polyzygotic multiple pregnancies has been observed in certain kindreds and races (e.g., up to 1/20 for blacks) suggesting the influence of an heritable factor. Monozygotic multiple pregnancies are independent of race or heredity. Polyzygotic multiple pregnancies are known to be associated with

*zygote - sperm + ovum until 1st division*
*Polyzygotic Twins - more common in blacks*
*Monozygotic Twins - independent of race*

*Twin-Twin Transfusion - recipient has worse prognosis, 70% mortality rate. CHF*

**98**     OB/GYN NOTES

states of gonadotropic overstimulation, the most common being iatrogenic (HMG/HCG or clomiphene-induced ovulation).

## Twins

Dizygotic twins account for 75% of twins and as explained they arise from the fertilization of two separate ova (released during one ovarian cycle) by two separate spermatozoa. Although each dizygotic twin always has its own chorion (and subsequently placenta), this may not be apparent if they have implanted close together. Nevertheless upon close inspection the circulations of the two fetuses are always separate.

Monozygotic twins account for the other 25% of twins. Such twins share a single placenta but possess individual amniotic sacs unless the latter breakdown during the course of pregnancy. If this does occur there is an increased risk of locking. Because the two fetuses share a single placenta, their circulatory system is also shared permitting one fetus the ability to monopolize the blood flow. This results in one fetus being smaller than the other despite identical genomes. The donor twin does not experience later "catch-up" growth. If arteriovenous malformations form within the placenta an exaggerated form of the above situation can occur, referred to as the *twin transfusion syndrome*. The donor is not only smaller for gestational age he or she is also anemic (Hb~80g/l) at birth; conversely the recipient is plethoric (Hb~270g/l) at birth. Donors may also have oligohydramnios if the integrity of the amniotic sac is preserved. Nonetheless it is the recipient neonate whose prognosis is worse. They are macrosomic, may have polyhydramnios and suffer congestive heart failure with an overall mortality rate approaching 70%.

## Superfetation Versus Superfecundation

Superfetation refers to the fertilization of two ova released during successive ovarian cycles. It is controversial whether this can actually occur as it is widely accepted that pregnancy suppresses ovulation. Superfecundation is the fertilization of two simultaneously released ova on two separate occasions (most easily diagnosed if the paternal genetic contribution is varied on each occasion).

*US at 18 wks*

### Diagnosis of Multiple Pregnancy. Suspicions of multiple pregnancy may

be raised in patients with positive family histories. Other suggestive features include: (1) excessive maternal weight gain; (2) exaggerated symptoms of pregnancy (e.g., hyperemesis gravidarum); (3) palpation of more than one head or breech; and (4) preterm labor. Sonographic or radiographic (after 18 weeks' gestation) confirmation should be sought.

The mother is at increased risk for PIH, polyhydramnios, anemia, and excessive weight gain. The infant is at increased risk of intrauterine growth retardation, malpresentation, congenital malformation, and early neonatal death (related chiefly to preterm delivery). The second and successive siblings are at increased risk of asphyxia and, therefore, of operative delivery. The labor process may also be affected with increased likelihood of PROM, umbilical cord prolapse, postpartum hemorrhage (uterine overdistension), and cervical incompetence.

The most common fetal presentations, in descending order of frequency for twins are:

- **Cephalic** : Cephalic
- **Cephalic** : Breech
- **Breech** : Breech

When the process that results in the formation of monozygous twins (division of the blastoderm) is incomplete, the resultant twins will share body parts. The resultant fetuses are referred to as **conjoined twins.** They are exceedingly rare in North America, $1/10^5$ live births (or 1/1000 twins). The etiology is unknown. Antepartum diagnosis is only achieved in 50% of cases. This can be accomplished by ultrasound when it is noted that the sonographic images of the twins cannot be separated or plain radiography reveals unusually close spines that do not change position relative to one another even after fetal movement.

Antepartum diagnostic success is poor, thus in any twin labor during which dystocia is encountered one must consider: (1) locking of the twins (one fetus impedes the descent and delivery of the other, e.g., breech/cephalic presentation); (2) major congenital anomaly; and (3) conjoined twins. Cesarean section is indicated for all conjoined twins except craniopagus.

## Triplets    *30% neonatal mortality*

For unknown reasons there is an increased incidence of female fetuses in triplet pregnancy. The presentation of the firstborn of a triplet is cephalic in the majority of cases, however, subsequent fetuses present by the breech as often as they do by the vertex of the head. Neonatal mortality approaches 30% but the following factors favor survival: (1) greater maternal age, (2) female fetus, (3) degree of fetal maturity, and (4) being born earlier once the labor process has commenced.

## GESTATIONAL TROPHOBLASTIC DISEASE    *80% Benign*

Gestational trophoblastic disease (GTD) covers a range of neoplastic disorders of the placenta or trophoblast including benign hydatidiform mole, locally invasive chorioadenoma destruens (CD), and frankly malignant and almost always metastatic choriocarcinoma (CC). Eighty percent of lesions initially diagnosed as moles follow a benign course, whereas 15% become locally invasive and 5% eventually become frankly malignant. Note that CC of GTD differs from the choriocarcinoma of the ovary (a germ cell tumor) in that the former is always associated with a pregnancy, whereas the latter is not.

The incidence of GTD varies greatly throughout the world being ~1 per 2000 pregnancies in North America, but much higher in Southeast Asia approaching 1 per 100 pregnancies in Taiwan. The incidence has also been noted to be higher in lower socioeconomic classes. The etiology is unknown, however, chromosomal aberration and nutritional deficiencies (e.g., folate) have been implicated.

*Folate deficiency*

## Hydatidiform Mole

Grossly edematous chorionic villi resembling **grapelike** structures are seen to involve all or any portion of the placenta. It is not unusual for the curettings from an individual with a molar pregnancy to appear grossly normal if only a fraction of the placenta is involved. A distinction should be made between **molar pregnancy** and **hydropic degeneration** of an otherwise normal pregnancy. A true mole is characterized by: (1) the absence of fetal tissue, (2) proliferation of the trophoblastic lining, (3) lack of blood vessels in the villi, and (4) marked edema of the villi. Hydatidiform mole is a benign neoplastic (proliferative) disorder, whereas hydropic degeneration is a degenerative process. Although villi that have undergone hydropic degeneration also appear grossly edematous they are not associated with trophoblastic proliferation; fetal tissue is present and degenerated villi exhibit a triploid chromosomal complement. The fetuses often have gross congenital anomalies. Conversely there is strongly suggestive evidence that molar pregnancies represent a duplication of spermatic genome without contribution from the ova.

## Chorioadenoma Destruens

_extensive local invasion of the endometrium_

Chorioadenoma destruens, like moles, are characterized by trophoblastic proliferation with preservation of the villous pattern, however, they also display extensive local invasion of the endometrium. The chief form of morbidity is hemorrhage due to infiltration of the adjacent blood vessels. On occasion metastatic lesions are found but they are well differentiated and regress spontaneously or are readily controlled by medical therapy.

## Choriocarcinoma

Choriocarcinoma is a very rare form of GTD (1/40,000 pregnancies in North America), but it is highly malignant and has often metastasized by the time it is detected. CC can be associated with any form of pregnancy; 50% have been observed to follow molar pregnancies (although only 5% of moles progress to choriocarcinoma), 30% with spontaneous abortions, and 20% follow apparently normal pregnancy (poor prognostic group).

Grossly choriocarcinoma may appear as a dark hemorrhagic mass on the surface of the uterus or vagina with or without ulceration. Uterine perforation with severe hemorrhage is relatively common. Benign trophoblast seldom extends beyond the venous system being limited by the pulmonary vasculature, however, malignant tumor emboli can extend beyond the pulmonary capillaries. Hemorrhage into a cerebral metastasis is not an uncommon mode of death. Marked occlusion of pulmonary vascular channels can cause pulmonary hypertension and cor pulmonale.

Microscopically there is total disorganization with loss of the villous pattern and proliferation extending into the adjacent muscular tissues. Histologic differentiation between benign and malignant lesions is based on the presence of muscle necrosis and the extent of invasion of adjacent tissue. The lesion is considered benign if the former is absent and the latter is limited to invasion by single cell or small cell groups; if muscle necrosis exists and the extent of invasion of underlying tissue is greater than small groups of cells, then the lesion is said to be malignant.

*Clinical Manifestations of GTD.* Clinically GTD presents before the 20th week of gestation with exaggerated signs and symptoms of pregnancy: hyperemesis gravidarum, preeclampsia (otherwise rare this early in pregnancy), thyrotoxicosis, and vaginal bleeding classically with the passage of grapelike edematous chorionic villi and uterine cramping. Intra-abdominal uterine perforation with massive blood loss presents as acute circulatory failure. The uterus is usually LGA (50%), but can be normal size (20%) or even SGA (30%). Malignant forms of the disease can present with metastatic manifestations either pulmonary (hemoptysis and cough), CNS (syndrome of space occupying lesions or intracerebral hemorrhage), or local metastases (vulvovaginal venous thromboses). Choriocarcinoma tends to metastasize early to lung, brain, liver, and bone.

Associated ovarian changes occur as a result of excess HCG stimulation and manifests in 20% of GTD as bilateral theca lutein cysts, which may later progress to ovarian malignancy. Similar cysts can, however, arise in normal pregnancy and may not appear until after evacuation of GTD. If appropriate therapy is undertaken for GTD, the ovarian changes will regress.

*Investigations.* In the presence of a LGA uterus with early (<20 week) gestational vaginal hemorrhage one should strongly suspect molar pregnancy. An inappropriately elevated serum beta-HCG level is supportive. HCG normally peaks toward the end of the first trimester. Multiple gestation is a benign cause for elevated beta-HCG levels but is almost never in excess of $10^5$ IU/L. Twenty-four-hour urine collections for HCG quantitation are obsolete. The typical sonographic appearance is described as the **"snowstorm"** or **"honeycomb"** pattern (a representation of the abnormal placental proliferation). Local metastases may be detected by pelvic examination but failing this, pelvic sonography or abdominopelvic angiography may be required. Chest x-ray (CXR) is sufficient to detect probable lung spread and hepatic ultrasound for hepatic involvement.

*Management.* Once the diagnosis of GTD is conclusively established, suction curettage is the treatment of choice. If preservation of reproductive capacity is not desired hysterectomy may be performed, however, suction curettage has been found to be the safest method of treatment. Trophoblastic pulmonary emboli have resulted both with hysterectomy and attempts to evacuate the uterus by induction of labor. Following evacuation of patients 80% resume normal menses, 15% develop CD, and 5% go on to have frank choriocarcinoma.

The postpartum serum beta-HCG level is an important marker of disease activity, therefore, repeat pregnancy must be avoided for at least 1 year. Beta-HCG values usually return to normal within 8 to 12 weeks of uterine evacuation but patients who develop malignancy may exhibit abnormally high beta-HCG levels as early as the fourth postevacuation week.

When the beta-HCG is negative for 4 weeks the patient is considered disease-free. She may then be seen monthly for 1 year for repeat assays, pelvic examination, and to detect any aberrations of menstrual function that might suggest recurrence. After 1 year of disease free follow-up no further investigation is warranted. Although repeat molar pregnancy has been reported, it is rare.

Malignant GTD usually presents clinically as vaginal hemorrhage after adequate uterine evacuation. Tissue diagnosis is not required if beta-HCG levels are elevated. Repeat evacuation (D & C) is required only to remove the source of hemorrhage.

Staging investigations generally include basic blood work (CBC, platelet count, liver, and renal function tests) and chest x-ray as well as other radiographic procedures (thoracic and cranial computed tomographic scan, liver and pelvic sonography, radionuclide bone scan). Abdominopelvic angiography is only rarely required. Both the duration of disease before diagnosis and the actual quantitative value of the beta-HCG are proportional to the likelihood of poor outcome. Other poor prognostic features may include

Progn. Factors

(1) Duration
(2) Quant. βHCG
(3) Prior failed chemo
(4) pp GTD @ Term Preg.

> Methotrexate
> Actinomycin - D
>
> CNS + Liver mets  unresponsive
> RT resistant

prior failed chemotherapy (50% mortality) and postpartum GTD after term pregnancy (40% mortality).

Chemotherapy is significantly more effective than other forms of oncotherapy. Indications for chemotherapy are:

1. Histologic diagnosis of choriocarcinoma
2. Documented metastases
3. Beta-HCG levels that:
   a. plateau or increase after uterine evacuation
   b. have not become negative after 12 weeks after uterine evacuation
   c. recurrent rise sometime after having been negative

The chief chemotherapeutic agents currently in use for malignant GTD are **methotrexate** (dihydrofolate acid reductase inhibitor) and **dactinomycin** (DNA-dependent RNA-polymerase antagonist). Although very efficacious for nonmetastatic disease neither of these agents crosses the blood–brain barrier and both are relatively rapidly metabolized by the liver thus making CNS and hepatic mets relatively resistant. Single agent therapy is employed for nonmetastatic disease and for those with low risk metastases, otherwise combination chemotherapy is indicated.

This form of malignancy is relatively radiotherapy-resistant. Hysterectomy is becoming less important in the management of malignant GTD. Indications for surgery include:

Surgery {
1. Drug resistance or toxicity
2. Persistent vaginal hemorrhage
3. Uterine perforation with intraperitoneal bleed
}

**Outcome.** Malignant GTD is very sensitive to methotrexate and dactinomycin (if they can gain access to the lesions), thus nonmetastatic disease has almost a 100% cure rate with single agent therapy, whereas high-risk metastatic disease with triple therapy has a lesser success rate. Chemotherapy is continued for one course after the beta-HCG reverts to negativity and the patient should be followed semi-annually for the next 2 years.

Good Prog Factors
1. Short duration (last preg w/in 4mos)
2. Pretx hCG < 40,000
3. No brain or liver mets
4. No signif. prior chemo tx

Poor Prog.
1. long duration (>4mos)
2. high Pretx hCG
3. ⊕ brain/liver mets
4. signif. prior chemo
5. Term Preg.

# OBSTETRIC MORTALITY

This section lists the specific definitions of certain terms used in the case of deaths associated with pregnancy as well as the reasons for the declining obstetric mortality in North America.

- *Birth:* The complete expulsion or extraction of a fetus from the mother regardless of whether or not the umbilical cord is severed or the placenta attached.
- *Live Birth:* Any infant that shows evidence of spontaneous respiration, cardiac activity, or movement of voluntary muscles or other signs of life after birth.
- *Abortus:* A fetus or embryo expelled or extracted from the uterus during the first half of gestation ($\leq 20$ weeks LMP), or weighing less than 500 g, or measuring less than 25 cm in length.
- *Fetal Death (stillbirth):* Infants showing no evidence of life (see above) after expulsion from the uterus.
- *Fetal Death Rate:* The number of fetal deaths per 1000 infants born.
- *Neonatal Mortality Rate:* The number of deaths of live-born infants during the first 28 days after birth per 1000 live births.
- *Perinatal Mortality Rate:* The number of fetal deaths plus neonatal deaths per 1000 total births.

- *Maternal Mortality Rate:* The number of maternal deaths that occur as a direct result of the reproductive process **per 100,000 live-births.**

The leading causes of maternal death are hemorrhage (35%), hypertensive disorders (25%), and infection (20%). The decline in maternal mortality over the past half century is attributed to the use of blood transfusion, better antihypertensive agents, and antibiotics, as well as better training of attending obstetric personnel.

The two leading causes of neonatal mortality include low birth weight (<2.5 kg) and CNS injury (whether due to obstetric trauma or ischemic/hypoxic insult). Improvements in neonatal survival are largely attributable to the techniques and knowledge that comprise a medical specialty that did not exist 50 years ago, neonatology.

# 4

# General Gynecology

## VULVAR DISEASES

### Inflammatory Disorders

Local irritants (vaginal discharge, urine, menstrual fluids) retained for prolonged intervals by tight, nonporous, synthetic undergarments contribute to
the relatively high incidence of inflammatory disorders of the vulva. General
prophylactic measures include: (1) loose cotton undergarments, (2) use of
nonperfumed drying agents, and (3) attentive perineal toilet (Table 4-1).

### Ulcerative Disorders

Ulcerative lesions induced by local trauma are nonspecific in appearance.
The accompanying discomfort is usually minimal and self-limiting. Prophylactic use of an antiseptic agent is sometimes suggested because of the
compromised integrity of the skin. Rarely such lesions may be self-inflicted
to avoid coitus.

　　Although usually an idiopathic disorder of young men, Behçet's syndrome may present in women as well. Behçet's syndrome is a triad of severe
anterior uveitis (iridocyclitis), oral ulcers, and genital ulcers. Behçet's syndrome may be associated with evidence of systemic vasculitis (e.g., thrombophlebitis, peripheral neuropathy) as well as synovitis. The cause of Behçet's syndrome is not known but there is evidence to suggest an underlying
autoimmune process. Therapy usually involves glucocorticoids or immu-
nosuppressants. Death can result from extensive central nervous system
(CNS) involvement.

*Behcets = autoimmune* **107**

**TABLE 4-1. INFLAMMATORY DISORDERS OF THE VULVA**

| Disorder | Etiology | Clinical | Comments | Treatment |
|---|---|---|---|---|
| Intertrigo | Persistent maceration | Crural/interlabial folds; Initially, erythematous, then linear fissuring; end stage, thick hyperkeratotic skin | Common wherever moist folds of integument are apposed; end stage often mistaken for "leukoplakia" | Drying powders; eliminate tight undergarments; fluorinated topical steroids. General measures listed in text |
| Seborrheic keratitis | Idiopathic excess sebaceous gland secretion | Crushed, scaling skin; becomes pruritic if chronic | | |
| Reactive dermatitis | Nuisance irritant provokes excessive self-inflicted manual maceration | Erythemia, heat, swelling, pain and evidence of the initiating process | Visible lesions are self inflicted; underlying cause of pruritis often not initially apparent | Careful history and physical exam to detect the initial cause; general measures and eliminate cause if identified |
| Psoriasis | Unknown | Round or ovoid patches of silver scales on erythematous base +/− linear excoriations | Rarely isolated to vulva | Topical steroids |
| Candidiasis | Candida species (notably C. albicans) | Usually vulvovaginal; beefy red base with tenacious white plaques; satellite lesions of papules and pustules on similar base | Most common vulvar infection; often associated with OCP, broad-spectrum antibiotic therapy, or Diabetes mellitus | Initially either nystatin, clotrimazole, or miconazole for 7–10 day and 2–3 day premenses & postmenses; for recurrences add 1% gentian violet to 7 day of any of the above |

**OCP,** oral contraceptive pill.

Regional enteritis may present with isolated perineal ulceration but more commonly there are associated sinus tracts or fistulae. Dermatologic signs may precede gastrointestinal or rheumatologic manifestations. Management of inflammatory bowel disease may involve systemic steroid therapy.

## Circulatory Diseases

Vulvar varices are relatively common. They are usually on the labia majora. Vulvar varices are the female equivalent of a varicoceles (varix of the pampiniform plexus) but unlike varicoceles they do not lead to infertility. Any process or condition associated with increased endopelvic pressure (pregnant uterus, a benign ovarian cyst, pelvic malignancy) can cause vulvar varices. They present as multiple, small superficial purple blood filled elevations that become more visible when standing or coughing.

Systemic ECF excess commonly manifests as grossly apparent edema at the vulva because of the relative insufficiency of skeletal support for vulvar adipose tissue and the dependency of the vulva. Vulvar edema can also result from local inflammatory disorders or lymphedema due to neoplastic, or infectious occlusion of regional lymphatic drainage. Prolonged unexplained edema should prompt consideration of pelvic mass lesion.

## White Lesions

White lesions may result from depigmentation or hyperkeratosis and include malignant neoplasms (Fig. 4-1).

Dystrophy is defined as any disorder due to defective tissue nutrition which may cause atrophy or hyperplasia. The classic form of vulvar atrophy is *lichen sclerosis atrophicus* (**LSA**). LSA is a postmenopausal disorder that initially manifests as a collection of small bluish white vulvar papules that coalesce to form a diffuse whitish area over the entire perineum. Subsequently, a cicatricial retraction causes flattening of the labia and "kraurosis" or shrinkage of the introitus. LSA can be intensely pruritic but is usually asymptomatic until the end-stage fibrosis causes dyspareunia. Biopsy is indicated to rule out malignant transformation (rare). Antipruritics and topical estrogen preparations are effective therapy. If biopsy and histologic examination reveal malignancy, vulvectomy may be warranted.

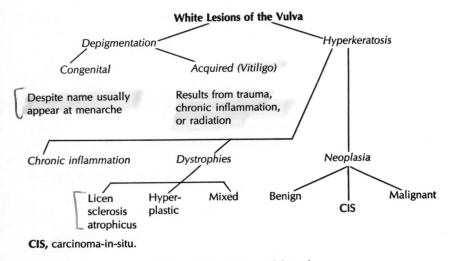

CIS, carcinoma-in-situ.

**Figure 4-1.** White lesions of the vulva.

Hyperplasia is defined as a focal increase in the number of cells within a tissue. Histologic abnormalities in the basal cell layer of the epithelium may warrant designation as an atypical form of hyperplasia. Atypical hyperplasia may be malignant or pre-malignant and therefore warrants biopsy.

## Glandular Disorders
Table 4-2 details the diagnostic signs and symptoms, as well as the treatment for glandular disorders of the vulva.

## Sexually Transmitted Diseases
Table 4-3 details the diagnostic signs and symptoms, as well as the treatment of the viral sexually transmitted diseases and Table 4-4 describes those of the bacterial form. Table 4-5 gives signs and symptoms of treponemal sexually transmitted diseases of the vulva.

**TABLE 4-2. GLANDULAR DISORDERS OF THE VULVA**

| Disorder | Clinical | Treatment |
|---|---|---|
| Major vestibular gland adenitis (acute bartholinitis) | Swollen, firm, painful with purulent exudate commonly proceeding to abscess; associated edema of labium majus may be very pronounced; most common cause is *N. gonorrheae* | Bedrest, icepacks, Sitz baths, analgesia; antimicrobial as per Table 4-3; if abscessed then incise and drain |
| Chronic bartholinitis | Above process may persist for years to form small nodules at 5 and 7 o'clock positions on labium majus; intermittently symptomatic; Cystic degeneration results from obstruction to drainage | For recurrent infection, excise gland; for cyst, marsupialize |
| Minor vestibular gland adenitis | Erythema dyspareunia | Often resistant to general measures; can be mistaken for neoplasia |
| Apocrine sweat gland adenitis (hydradenitis) | Seen also at axillary vault; mild, recurrent purulent pustules; Severe, suppuration resembling folliculitis; extensive tissue damage; draining sinuses; lymphedema/adenopathy | General measures; OCP's decrease apocrine secretions; rarely surgical debridement |
| Fox-Fordyce disease | Same as above but with intense pruritus and focal dilatation of the glands giving rise to multiple fine vulvar papules | Same as above |

**OCP,** oral contraceptive pill.

**TABLE 4-3. SEXUALLY TRANSMITTED DISEASES (VIRAL)**

| Disorder | Etiology | Clinical | Comments/Treatment |
|---|---|---|---|
| Herpes genitalis (occasionally HSV$_1$) | HSV$_2$ | Initially asymptomatic vesicles; breakdown to painful superficial serpiginous ulcers; extensive labial edema, tenderness, and inguinal adenopathy; +/− possible systemic complaints (fever, malaise); vagina/cervix may be involved | Prone to secondary bacterial infection; serology not helpful, too many seropositive asymptomatics; characteristic multinucleated giant cells and intranuclear inclusions; bedrest, 5% acyclovir x6/d for 7d; cesarean section if infection active during third trimester |
| Condyloma accuminatum (pointy warts) | Unknown (HPV) | Multiple discrete warts on thighs, perineum, vagina, cervix, and perianally; tend to confluence and hypertrophy during pregnancy; regress spontaneously postpartum | Associated with trichomonal and candidal infection as well as OCP; cryotherapy, topical 5-fluorouracil or 20% podophyllin |
| Molluscum contagiosum | Papilloma virus Measles | Pearly white umbilicated papules; usually asymptomatic | Rarely warrant therapy |

**char,** characteristic; **d,** day(s); **OCP,** oral contraceptive.

## Urethral Diseases

Urethritis, in the sexually active woman, is most commonly **gonococcal,** although **chlamydia** is increasing in incidence. Gonococcus usually causes cervicitis and infrequently vaginitis (prepubertal, postmenopausal). In women the symptoms are usually evanescent but the process commonly persists into chronicity involving Skene's ducts and the periurethral glands. Nongonococcal urethritis in women is usually due to chlamydial or gram negative bacterial infection. Treatment with tetracycline or erythromycin for the former and with sulfas or ampicillin for the latter is usually sufficient. Chronic infection may respond to topical $AgNO_3$.

Postmenopausal urethritis is usually an aseptic process due to chemical irritation of atrophic urethral epithelium. Estrogen insufficiency weakens the surface epithelium. The urethra appears reddened and edematous and may even prolapse to mimic caruncles. The patient may complain of strangury and hematuria. Topical estrogen preparations are usually adequate therapy.

Chronic urethral inflammation can lead to stricture formation requiring surgical dilatation.

## Neoplastic Disorders

Carcinoma-in-situ, defined as full thickness epithelial replacement by undifferentiated cells without breaching the integrity of the underlying basement membrane, is rarely found in vulvar neoplasm. CIS occurs in only two distinct forms despite the three names (Tables 4-6 to 4-8). The first two, **Bowen's disease** and **erythroplasia of Queyrat** were initially believed to be different entities but microscopically they appear to be the same.

**Paget's disease of the vulva** is a distinct entity from both Paget's disease of bone or Paget's disease of the breast. Paget's disease of the vulva is a rare multifocal form of CIS that occurs during the perimenopausal years. Clinically it appears as focal gray–white patches on a reddish base. When CIS is documented, the therapeutic intervention of choice is either wide local excision or simple vulvectomy.

Malignant vulvar disease is invariably a disease of elderly women, usually the seventh decade. In the presence of chronic inflammatory processes, such as chronic granulomatous infections, the mean age of presentation is lower, ($\sim$40 years of age). The histologic types, listed in order of

**TABLE 4-4. SEXUALLY TRANSMITTED DISEASES (BACTERIAL)**

| Disorder | Etiology | Clinical |
|---|---|---|
| Granuloma inguinale | *Calymmatobacterium granulomatis* (Donovan bodies) | Incubation variable from days to months; initially small papules on labia minora then serpiginous ulcer on red granular base with purulent exudate; less painful than chancroid; Bx to R/O TB or malignancy; dark field to R/O syphilis |
| Lymphogranuloma venereum | *Chlamydia trachomatis*[a] | Incubation several days; initial lesion is evanescent papule or pustule (vaginal, cervical, or vulvar), then suppurative inguinal buboes; lymphedema; draining sinuses; fever and malaise; finally may result in endopelvic organ involvement with rectal and urethral strictures |
| Chancroid | *Hemophilus ducreyi* | 2–3 d incubation; papule/pustule with progression to indurated, painful ulcer; labia edema |

[a]*Chlamydia trachomatis* may also cause an uncomplicated urethritis as an STD; treat with Tc or Em 0.25g PO QID x21d.
**#1**, first drug of choice; **#2**, second drug of choice; **Bx**, biopsy; **CF**, compliment fixation;

frequency are: squamous cell, basal cell, melanoma, and sarcoma. Squamous cell lesions grossly may be ulcerative, white plaques, or fungating. Basal cell carcinoma of the vulva may present as "rodent" ulcers, i.e., ulcers with rolled edges. Squamous cell and basal cell carcinomas metastasize late. Simple vulvectomy may represent sufficient treatment. Malignant

| Laboratory | Comments | Treatment |
|---|---|---|
| 80% of plain smears pos for "safety pin" shaped **Donovan** inclusions; ~99%-Wright/Giemsa stain sensitivity | Adenopathy is rare; tends to remain superficial; extragenital sites, bone and skin | #1 Tc; #2 Sm; if chronic may require Sx; extragenital may be fatal Tc, 0.25–0.50 g PO q6h x14d Sm, 0.50–2.0 g IM OD x14d |
| Culture; Friel skin test; CF serology; Bx may show pseudotubercles | Essentially an STD of the lymphatics; nodes are either indurated ulcers or hypertrophic buboes; extragenital spread to bowel or meninges possible | Must Bx to R/O malignancy then #1 Tc or Em; #2 Cm; local infection self-limiting but extragenital sites persist without treatment Tc or Em, 0.50 g PO QID x21d Cm, 50 mg/kg/d PO as q6h x21d |
| *H. ducreyi* demonstrable on plain smear | Nonsuppurative inguinal adenitis common; coital transmission only | Good response to local antiseptic and #1 TMP/SMX; #2 Em TMP/SMX, 160 mg/ 800 mg PO BID x5d Em, 0.50 g PO QID x7d |

**Cm**, chloramphenicol; **d**, day; **Em**, erythromycin; **Pos**, positive; **R/O**, rule out; **Sm**, streptomycin; **STD**, sexually transmitted disease; **Sx**, surgery; **Tc**, tetracycline; **TMP/SMX**, cotrimoxazole

melanoma, though not common tends to metastasize early to regional lymph nodes in both groins.

Patients usually present with complaints of pruritus or ulceration. There is often a 1.5- to 2-year delay in presentation, due in combination to patient reluctance and the frequent absence of symptoms. Biopsy is mandatory for

**TABLE 4-5. TREPONEMAL STDS OF THE VULVA (*TREPONEMA PALLIDUM*)**

| Stage | Clinical | Lab | Comments/Treatment |
|---|---|---|---|
| Primary | Chancre, indurated indolent ulcer; +/− labium majus edema; marked inguinal adenitis; incubation 3–4 wk, self-limited in 4–6 wk | Dark field micro from ulcer; VDRL not reliable until secondary stage | Less apparent in women; if Tx'ed prior to 18th wk gestation prevents fetal infection; DOC is Pen G  ~~2.4 million u  X1 IM~~ |
| Secondary | Condyloma latum (flat warts), raised rounded indurated plateaulike lesions +/− gray necrotic exudate (thighs, perineum/perianal) generalized maculopapular rash with lymphadenitis | VDRL | Rash involves both palms and soles, may be tender; most infective stage of syphilis; onset > 6 wk after primary stage ends; DOC is Pen G |
| Tertiary | 70% are asymptomatic; 15% have classical gummatous lesions but they usually ulcerate; sloughing with perineal fistulae; 15% have CVS or CNS lesions | False-negative VDRL up to 33%; FTA-abs, TPI required to R/O Dx | CVS = obliterative end arteritis with luetic aortitis; tabes dorsalis = a triad of luetic aortitis, loss of posterior columns, and neurogenic joint; Other CNS forms include GPI and meningovascular forms; DOC is still Pen G |

**Early** (primary, secondary, or latent for < 1 yr): benzathine Pen G 2.4 million units IM once.

**Late** (>1 yr duration or cardiovascular system involvement) 2.4 million units IM weekly x3.

**Neurosyphilis:** Crystalline Pen G 2–4 million units IV q4h x10d or procaine Pen G 2.4 million units IM OD plus probenicid 0.50 g PO QID both x10d or benzathine Pen G 2.4 million units IM weekly x3; Tc or Em 0.50 g PO QID as alternatives to Pen G for 15d for **early** but for 30d for **late and neurosyphilis.**

CVS, cardiovascular system; DOC, drug of choice; Dx, diagnosis; Em, erythromycin; FTA-abs, fluorescent treponemal antibody (absorbed) test; GPI, general paresis of the insane; Micro, microscopy; Pen G, penicillin G; R/O, rule out; Tc, tetracycline; TPI, *Treponema pallidum* inhibition test; Tx'ed, treated; VDRL, venereal diseases reseach laboratories

**TABLE 4-6. NEOPLASTIC DISORDERS OF THE VULVA**

| Benign | | Malignant | |
|---|---|---|---|
| *Cystic* | *Solid* | *CIS* | *Invasive* |
| Bartholin duct | Fibroma | Bowen's disease | Squamous cell ca |
| Sebaceous | Lipoma | Erythroplasia of Queyrat | Basal cell ca |
| Mucinous | Angioma | Paget's disease | Melanoma |
| Gartner's duct ⎤ | Hidradenoma | | Sarcoma |
| Nuck's canal ⎦ | Nevus | | |
| Endometriosis | Granular cell | | |
| | Myoblastoma | | |

**Ca,** carcinoma; **Gartner's duct** = Wolffian duct; **Nuck's canal** = processuss vaginalis (cyst of Nuck's canal is the female equivalent of a hydrocele).

any suspicious lesion. Eradication of chronic inflammatory processes may prevent malignancy from developing. Radical vulvectomy is indicated for all invasive disease with the exception perhaps of basal cell carcinoma.

## Leukoplakia and Pruritus Vulvae

One final note about two frequently misused terms. Leukoplakia is often misused to denote a white vulvar lesion with some particular significance. This is erroneous. The term simply means any white lesion.

Pruritus vulvae is often misused in the same way when in fact it is a generic term that implies no particular etiology. Therapy includes elimination of local irritants and antipruritic agents. Topical estrogens are only helpful if the problem is due to epithelial atrophy, otherwise topical androgenic preparations are advised. Subcutaneous injections of 95% alcohol may be used if other measures fail. Relief of pruritus is important because the chronic irritation of scratching may promote more sinister disease.

## VAGINAL DISEASES

Two basic disease processes affect the vagina inflammation (vaginitis) (Table 4-9) and neoplasia (Fig. 4-2). Inflammatory disorders of the vagina are far more common than neoplastic disorders.

**TABLE 4-7. BENIGN CYSTIC VULVAR NEOPLASIA**

| Disorder | Clinical Appearance | Comments |
|---|---|---|
| Bartholin duct | See glandular disorders | |
| Sebaceous/inclusion cyst | Initially small papules containing cheesy material on inner surface of labia minora; prone to complication by suppurative infection; when chronic they develop a lining of stratified epithelium, then called inclusion cysts | Result from inflammatory blockage of sebaceous glands; no treatment required unless recurrent infection develops, then surgical excision |
| Mucinous cyst | Often pedunculated; found near urethra or inner surface labia minora | Represent dilated obstructed minor vestibular glands |
| Gartner's duct cyst | Rarely appear on vulva proper but may project beyond introitus from within vagina | |
| Nuck's canal cyst ("hydrocele") _inguinal canal_ | Present as a swelling at the point of insertion of the round ligament on labium majus | Anomaly of processus vaginalis |
| Endometriosis | Rarely seen on vulva; at Bartholin glands, along round ligament in inguinal canal; cyclic recurrence of a painful nodule | See pelvic pain section |

_leukorrhea — excessive vag discharge_

**TABLE 4-8. BENIGN SOLID VULVAR NEOPLASIA**

| Disorder | Clinical Appearance | Comments |
|---|---|---|
| Fibroma | Usually small pedunculated lesions; resemble myxomatous tissue microscopically | Surgical excision if large |
| Lipoma | Rarely seen here; similar to above in appearance | Excise if troublesome |
| Angioma | Congenital; rare; may irritate diapers | Regress spontaneously as child grows; no treatment required |
| Hidradenoma | Rare but often mistaken for adenocarcinoma; small nodule covered with red, granular, friable skin on inner surface of labia majora | Arise from vulvar sweat glands; usually benign |
| Nevus | May become malignant; flat expanding lesions most suspect; vulva represents 1% of SA but 4% of melanomas found here | Biopsy all pigmented lesions |
| Granular cell myoblastoma | Rare tumor usually seen in tongue; arises from myelin sheath; overlying pseudoepitheliomatous changes commonly mistaken for squamous cell carcinoma | |

SA, surface area.

The vaginitides are rarely life threatening disorders but they tend to recur due to cyclic variations in the hormonally governed composition of the vaginal epithelium. Vaginitides are usually infectious, and the chief complaint is excessive vaginal discharge (leukorrhea). The two natural defense mechanisms against vaginal infection are: (1) the mechanical barrier of an intact estrogen supported vaginal epithelium, and (2) the presence of commensal vaginal microorganisms. The primary vaginal commensal is lactobacillus that acidifies (pH 4.5–5.0) vaginal mucous. The low pH inhibits the growth of pathogenic bacteria. Factors that predispose to vaginal infection include: (1) diabetes mellitus; (2) broad spectrum antibiotic therapy;

## TABLE 4-9. VAGINITIDES[a]

| Etiology | Clinical Appearance | Lab |
|---|---|---|
| *Trichomonas vaginalis* | Copious yellow/green foamy discharge; burning discomfort $+/-$ dyspareunia or dysuria; **"strawberry" petechial erosions on vaginal mucosa** | Plain smear suffices but without douche or lubricant |
| *Candida* species | **Intense pruritus**; cheesy discharge with intense vulvovaginal irritation and reddening | Mycelia and conidia visible on KOH preparation; culture for confirmation on Nickerson or Sabouraud media |
| *Gardnerella vaginalis* | **Foul-smelling discharge**; otherwise little or no discomfort or pruritus; "fishy" odor when KOH added | Plain smear may demonstrate microbe but also shows paucity of PMNs and lactobacilli; culture on Casman blood agar or thioglycolate broth |
| *Neisseria gonorrhoeae* | Persistent discharge; marked local irritation; if untreated will persist into chronicity until puberty when epithelium is strengthened by endogenous estrogen | Visualization of gram-negative intracellular "coffee-bean"-shaped organisms is only presumptive evidence; culture on Thayer–Martin in 10% $CO_2$ |
| Herpes simplex virus$_2$ | Tender, edematous mucosa with vesicles that breakdown to form serpiginous ulcers on red base; 2–3 d incubation | Multinucleated giant cells and acidophilic intranuclear inclusions |
| Postmenopausal | Thin blood-tinged discharge with pruritus and burning; $+/-$ stricture formation with dyspareunia | |
| Emphysematous | Gas-filled blebs in the submucosal layers of vagina | |

[a]These disorders are primarily sexually transmitted diseases.
**KOH**, potassium hydroxide; **Pen G,** *penicillin G*; **PMN**, polymorphonuclear leukocytes; **Tc**, tetracycline;

| Comments | Treatment |
|---|---|
| Common especially in pregnancy; often asymptomatic; primarily spread by sexual contact | Metronidazole, 0.5 g PO BID x7d or 2.0 g PO as single dose; picric acid suppositories lower pH, thus promote lactobacillus growth; during pregnancy, 20% NaCl douche (avoid iodine, may cause fetal thyroid suppression), or 2x 100 mg clotrimazole vaginal suppository QHS x7d |
| 10% incidence among nonpregnant, 33% if pregnant; also common postmenopausally; fomite and venereal spread | Miconazole or clotrimazole suppository intravaginally OD x7d or nystatin 100,000 units intravaginally QHS x14d (oral nystatin is not absorbed from GI tract and therefore ineffective) |
| **Clue cells** seen on smears are epithelial cells with gram-negative coccobacilli adherent to surface | Metronidazole, 0.50 g PO BID x7d or ampicillin, 0.50 g PO BID x7d |
| Only causes vaginitis when epithelium is thin (prepubertal and postmenopausal); may represent child abuse | Amoxicillin, 3.0 g PO once with 1.0 g PO probenicid followed by Tc, 0.50 g PO QID x7d or procaine Pen G, 4.8 million units IM plus 1.0 g PO probenicid once or spectinomycin, 2.0 g IM once or cefoxitin, 2.0 g or cefuroxime, 1.5 g IM each once plus probenicid as above or cefotaxime, 1.0 g IM once |
| Orogenital contact increases chance of HSV$_1$ herpes genitalis and HSV$_2$ herpes gingivitis | Acyclovir, 5% cream 6x/d x7d decreases duration of viral shedding during initial infection; less effective for recurrent infections |
| | Topical estrogen preparations 2–3x/wk then repeat once weekly to prevent recurrence |
| | **Emphysematous vaginitis** associated with pregnancy, congestive heart failure, and trichomonal infection, no treatment required |

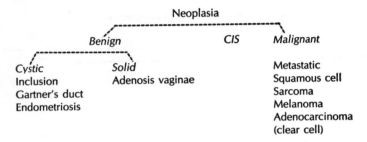

**Figure 4-2.** Vaginal neoplastic disorders.

(3) varicella zoster virus (VZV) infection in children; (4) foreign bodies (common in the pediatric age group); (5) oral contraceptive pill (OCP); and (6) pregnancy.

Inclusion cysts originate from ectopic mucosal epithelium trapped beneath the surface that becomes encysted in a lining of stratified squamous epithelium. They are more commonly found posteriorly or on the vaginal vault. Inclusion cysts are more common after perineal tears, episiotomies, and hysterectomies.

Gartner's duct cysts arise from the remnants of the mesonephric (Wolffian) system and are usually seen in the anterolateral aspect of the vaginal canal (see vulvar disorders).

Endometriosis is rarely a diffuse process in the vagina but can present at the vault as lesions penetrate from the pouch of Douglas. They appear as subepithelial nodules or hemorrhagic areas.

Adenosis vaginae refers to a roughened area of ectopic mucous secreting glands within the vagina. Adenosis vaginae occurs more frequently in women whose mothers took oral estrogen (e.g., diethylstilbestrol, DES) preparations during the course of their pregnancy. Fetal exposure to estrogens during genital tract formation may result in inferior displacement of the normal junction between the Müllerian system and the urogenital sinus. An otherwise rare malignancy, clear cell carcinoma of the vagina exhibits a higher incidence than expected in this population of women and may arise from such ectopic Müllerian remnants.

DES → clear cell Ca

Primary carcinomas of the vagina are rare. Squamous cell carcinoma tends to occur in the sixth decade. The incidence of adenocarcinoma or clear cell carcinoma peaks during the second to third decades. Sarcoma botryoides (very rare) usually presents before completion of the first decade. Squamous cell carcinoma accounts for 95% of primary vaginal malignancies and usually arises from the vaginal vault as a friable fungating mass or ulcerative lesion. Patients usually present with a bloody discharge or protruding mass. There is early spread to other pelvic organs. Sarcoma botryoides is a highly malignant multicentric lesion that usually presents as a grapelike pink edematous mass protruding from the introitus. Primary vaginal melanoma has a poor prognosis because it often escapes early detection.

Vaginal carcinoma-in-situ is multicentric, and therefore warrants total vaginectomy. Radiotherapy is less dysfiguring but can promote stricture formation and radiation induced vaginitis obscures further cytologic evaluation. Pelvic exenteration with bowel and bladder diversion is indicated for squamous cell carcinoma. Radiotherapy is often applied adjunctively. Sarcoma botryoides is so highly malignant that even total vaginectomy and hysterectomy do not alter the otherwise dismal prognosis.

## PELVIC PAIN (SECONDARY DYSMENORRHEA)

This discussion concerns itself with the potential gynecologic causes of pelvic pain in women (Table 4-10). The patient usually complains of pain localized to the suprapubic, iliac fossae, sacral, or medial thigh regions. Dyspareunia may also be the presenting complaint. The pain may be acute, with associated gastrointestinal (GI) complaints or chronic (episodic or low-grade persistent) with exacerbations during ovulation, menses, or intercourse. Although this section details only the potential gynecologic entities responsible for pelvic pain, one should also consider nongynecologic pathology, e.g., GI tract and urinary tract.

The most common gynecologic causes of pelvic pain are:

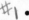

- Salpingitis (pelvic inflammatory disease, PID)
- Endometriosis

124

## TABLE 4-10. PELVIC PAIN

| Diagnosis | Timing | Clinical |
|---|---|---|
| Salpingitis | Onset often postpartum or postmenstrual | Pain and tenderness usually bilateral, acute, or chronic but generally progressive; fever; purulent discharge; unilateral symptoms with IUD; +/− nausea and vomiting |
| Ovulation hemorrhage | Sine qua non; mid-cycle of a normal ovulatory period | Evidence of intraperitoneal hemorrhage; shoulder pain, ↑ HR, ↓ BP, and abdominal distension; +/− vaginal bleeding due to postovulatory estrogen depletion |
| Adnexal torsion | Unpredictable | Acute, unilateral, severe pain with nausea/emesis; evidence of peritonism: abdominal wall tenderness, rebound tenderness, rigidity; +/− palpable mass |
| Endometriosis | Exacerbated with menses | Reported as a cramping, dull ache or bearing down sensation in low back or abdomen; dyspareunia suggests uterosacral/pouch of Douglas disease; dysuria suggests bladder involvement; aberrations of menstrual blood loss (DUB) suggests ovarian disease; hemoptysis at menses suggests pulmonary lesions; rectal bleed or obstruction suggests colonic disease; infertility; therapy induces amenorrhea until discontinued |
| Ectopic pregnancy | Follows menses by a time period greater than normal menstrual interval (usually < 8 wk LMP) | Evidence of intraperitoneal hemorrhage (listed above); pain is unilateral and severe becoming diffuse; acute implies isthmic nidation; subacute with ampullary nidation; evidence of peritonism (listed above); +/− vaginal bleed; ("funny pain, funny period") |

**Beta-HCG**, blood assay for beat subunit of human chorionic gonadotropin; **BP**, blood pressure; **C/S**, culture and sensitivity; **D & C**, dilatation and curettage; **DUB**, dysfunctional uterine bleeding; **GC**, gonococcus; **Hb**, hemoglobin; **HR**, heart rate; **IUD**, intrauterine

| Pelvic Examination | Lab | Treatment |
|---|---|---|
| Enlarged tender uterus; bloody/purulent discharge; tender adnexal masses; pelvic "heat"; signs of recent pregnancy if postpartal | Cervical C/S for GC, aerobic and anaerobic organisms; U/S; +/− laparoscopy with fallopian tube cultures; elevated WBC | Antibiotics according to C/S result; D & C if postpartal; USO/ BSO if extensive disease present; (see Table 4-11 for empiric therapy) |
| Normal uterus; diffuse tenderness; no masses; no pelvic "heat" | Culdocentesis; +/− laparoscopy; WBC not elevated; Hb ↓ variably | Fluid replacement; excise and oversew offending corpus luteum |
| Unilateral tender mass | ↑ WBC | Laparotomy with resection; do not untwist, may embolize |
| Multiple nodules posterior fornix (along uterosacral ligaments); enlarge and become more tender with menses; excitatory pain; adnexal nodularity or thickening | Laparoscopy to document extent of disease | Analgesics; hormonal with progestins, predominantly progestational OCPs or danazol, low dose androgens; Sx |
| Enlarged (50% with unilateral asymmetry); excitatory pain; no pelvic "heat" | Hb ↓ ; beta-HCG reverts to negativity or shows downward trend; U/S; culdocentesis; laparoscopy | Sx, see further notes |

device; **LMP**, last menstrual period; **OCP**, oral contraceptive pill; **pelvic heat and excitatory pain**, see salpingitis notes; **Sx**, surgery; **U/S**, ultrasound; **USO/BSO**, unilateral/bilateral salpingo-oopherectomy; **WBC**, white blood cell count; **+/−**, with or without.

- Ectopic pregnancy
- Adnexal torsion
- Ovulation hemorrhage (mittelschmerz)

Salpingitis, endometriosis, and ectopic pregnancy are discussed in greater detail.

## Salpingitis

The primary sites of pelvic inflammation are the fallopian tubes, hence the term salpingitis. The endometrium, ovaries and adjacent pelvic organs, and peritoneum may also be involved. PID is usually infectious in origin. Inoculation may result from upward migration from the vagina after sexual contact with an infected partner or hematogenous dissemination (*Mycobacterium tuberculosis*). Local genital acquisition is by far more common. The endometrium is normally protected by regular shedding during the menstrual cycle. Amenorrhea for any cause (e.g., pregnancy) increases the risk of endometrial and therefore fallopian infection. The clinical course is variable with either acute or chronic presentation.

### Etiology

- *Neisseria gonorrhoeae*
- Pyogenic organisms (gram-positive and gram-negative aerobes and gram-negative anaerobes)
- *Chlamydia* sp.
- *Mycoplasma* sp.
- *Mycobacterium tuberculosis*

Gonococcus is the most common cause. The initial cervicitis is commonly asymptomatic in women and therefore often presents late with disseminated gonococcemia or salpingitis or sterility or both.

Pyogenic salpingitis may in fact be a secondary phenomenon following primary gonococcal infection. The causative organisms include *Escherichia coli, Streptococcus viridans*, enterococcal streptococci, and *Bacteroides fragilis*. These organisms can rapidly destroy (extensive scarring) the genitourinary tract (GU), causing sterility.

*Chlamydia trachomatis* serotypes D through K, *Mycoplasma hominis*, and *Ureaplasma ureolyticum* (also designated T or Tiny strains of *Mycoplasma*) have recently been documented with increasing frequency. Improvements in the acquisition of culture samples obtained from the fimbriated edge of the oviducts by laparoscopy and better culture techniques for these particularly fastidious organisms have permitted their documentation. The mode of infection is venereal.

Salpingitis due to *Mycobacterium tuberculosis* infection is responsible for less than 5% of cases in North America. It is, nonetheless, significant because it is not sexually transmitted.

*Pathology.* The immediate focus of most GU tract infections in women of childbearing age is the cervix from which upward spread occurs usually during menses. An asymptomatic carrier state has been documented for all of the previously noted microorganisms. The characteristic clinical picture is only manifest when the salpinges becomes inflamed.

Endometritis occurs most often during the puerperium or postabortal period. Microscopically there is edema with polymorphonuclear (PMN) leukocytic infiltration and hyperemia. If there has been instrumentation, then uterine perforation with parametritis (inflammation of the broad ligaments) may occur. Pelvic thrombophlebitis is a rare complication of salpingitis. Tubal inflammation results from direct mucosal spread of infection from the cervix (during pregnancy lymphatic dissemination is also implicated) necessitating intercurrent endometrial involvement. Endometritis in this circumstance is usually transient due to the protective effect of regular menstrual sloughing.

Tubal inflammation may occur immediately after lower tract infection or it may be delayed while the organism proliferates asymptomatically on the cervix. Although menstrual flow occurs in an outward direction the remaining endometrium is denuded and, therefore, particularly vulnerable to infection. This may explain the temporal relationship between menses and de novo symptoms or exacerbations. Endometrial infection facilitates salpingitis and the onset of symptoms. If one or both ends of the fallopian tube become occluded a pyosalpinx (pus-filled tube) may develop. An untreated pyosalpinx often progresses to become a hydrosalpinx (permanently damaged serous fluid filled tube). Gonococcus usually causes an endo-salpingitis, whereas the secondary pyogenic agents cause transmural inflammation and even perisalpingitis. Resolution is accompanied by cicatrization resulting in dysfunctional tubes, often making the patient sterile.

Ovarian involvement usually takes the form of a perio-ophoritis but may abscess (tubo-ovarian abscess).

Adjacent peritoneal inflammation may result from pus exuding from the free end of the tube. Local peritonitis can be complicated by cul-de-sac abscess formation. Posterior colpotomy is sufficient for drainage provided this is known to be the only site of involvement. The sudden rupture of such an abscess can lead to acute generalization of the peritoneal process causing acute circulatory failure. Total abdominal hysterectomy with bilateral salpingo-oopherectomy (TAH/BSO) has decreased the mortality for pelvic abscess rupture from 90% to ~5%. Transmural salpingitis leads to adhesion formation further impairing tubal function. Salpingolysis is required to free the tubes of peritubal adhesions.

Fitz-Hugh Curtis syndrome is a rare form of perihepatitis resulting from gonococcal infection that migrates up the right paracolic gutter. Patients may present with fever, right upper quadrant pain, and tenderness and possibly a hepatic friction rub. Subsequent generalized peritonitis may ensue.

***Clinical.*** Pelvic vaginal examination must be carried out carefully to elicit the maximum amount of information possible (Table 4-10). Commencing with the speculum examination of the cervix, swabs should be taken for Gram stain and gonococcal (GC) aerobic and anaerobic culture (Thayer Martin medium in 10% $CO_2$). In the acute situation masses are rarely detectable and the digital examination is often limited by excitatory pain, i.e., marked tenderness on transvaginal manipulation of the uterus and adnexae. Pelvic "heat" is the expression used for palpable warmth secondary to inflammatory hyperemia. If rectal examination also reveals tenderness one should suspect pouch of Douglas extension.

***Diagnostic Considerations.*** Intracellular gram-negative diplococci are only presumptive evidence of gonococcal cervicitis and culture positivity is diagnostic only for GC, *Chlamydia, Mycoplasma,* and the anaerobes.

*Fitz-Hugh Curtis*

Pyogenic aerobes are part of the normal vaginal flora making this diagnosis one of exclusion. A history of prior venereal infection or sexual contact with an infected partner is helpful but is often difficult to elicit. Laparoscopy is presently indicated to rule out other potentially hazardous pathologic processes or when the diagnosis is in doubt. Routine culture of the fallopian tubes is not indicated.

Tubal inflammation usually causes bilateral disease except for rare cases associated with intrauterine devices (IUDs). An increased incidence of unilateral infection and rarely infection with actinomycosis is noted in this situation. The presentation is usually subacute. The infected IUD must be removed to ensure effective eradication of disease.

Acute pyelonephritis may be difficult to distinguish from salpingitis. The pain of pyelonephritis, however, is usually in the lumbar region with flank radiation and costovertebral angle (CVA) tenderness. Renal infection is commonly preceded by symptomatic cystitis. Urine cultures and urinalysis are suggested to document urinary tract infection.

Acute appendicitis must also be considered if the patient presents with unilateral right lower quadrant abdominal pain. Primary appendiceal inflammation can be complicated by salpingitis if the appendix is pelvic in location (~30%) further confusing the clinical presentation of these disorders. Pain due to appendiceal inflammation is initially generalized and only later localized (to McBurney's point), whereas with salpingitis the reverse is true. Cervical cultures are negative in appendicitis.

**Treatment.** General supportive management including bedrest, intravenous crystalloid, and analgesia should be provided in addition to antibiotic therapy. Initial empiric therapy must cover all the likely pathogens. The choice and dosage of antibiotics is governed by whether the patient can be effectively managed as an outpatient or not (Table 4-11).

If the response to conservative therapy is unsatisfactory one should suspect either an incorrect diagnosis or loculation of pus. Diagnostic laparoscopy is helpful in this setting. Posterior colpotomy may be attempted as a drainage procedure if a cul-de-sac abscess is suspected. If this proves unsatisfactory, excisional surgery may be performed. *Clostridium perfringens* is an unlikely pathogen except when septic abortion has preceded the illness. Persistent fluctuating fever after extirpative surgery is suggestive

*C. perfringens unlikely pathogen except when septic Ab precedes illness.*

**TABLE 4-11. EMPIRIC ANTIBIOTIC THERAPY FOR SALPINGITIS**

| Patient Status | Drug Regimen | Comments |
|---|---|---|
| Outpatient | 1. CFX 2.0 g IM with probenecid 1.0 g PO once followed by doxycycline 100 mg PO BID × 10 d | CFX covers GC, anaerobes, and aerobes; doxycycline covers Chlamydia and Mycoplasma |
| | 2. Tc 500 mg PO QID × 10 d | Tc can cover all the possible organisms but is C/I in pregnancy |
| | 3. Amp 3.5 g **or** amx 3.0 g PO **or** procaine pen G 4.8 MU IM with probenecid 1.0 g PO once followed by doxycycline 100 mg PO BID × 10 d | Amp/Amx/Pen G for GC (PPNG will persist) |
| Inpatient | 1. CFX 2.0 g IV QID with doxycycline 100 mg IV BID until improved, then doxycycline 100 mg PO BID to complete 10 d | |
| | 2. Doxycycline 100 mg IV BID with metro 1.0 g IV BID until improved, then doxycycline 100 mg PO BID with metro 1.0 g PO BID to complete 10 d | Metro for anaerobes instead of CFX |

**Amp,** ampicillin; **Amx,** amoxicillin; **CFX,** cefoxitin; **C/I,** contraindicated; **GC,** gonococcus; **Metro,** metronidazole; **MU,** megaunits; **Pen G,** penicillin G; **PPNG,** penicillinase-producing *Neisseria gonorrhoeae;* **Tc,** tetracycline.

of pelvic vein thrombophlebitis. Gonococcal and pyogenic infections tend to be more virulent, leaving more anatomic damage in their wake than *Chlamydia* or *Mycoplasma* infections, which are often self-limited.

## Chronic Salpingitis

Chronic salpingitis may cause low grade persistent or recurrent episodic symptoms. The chief complaints are pain or infertility, or both.

*Pathology.* The microscopic pathology is unremarkable resembling that of chronic inflammation seen elsewhere. Grossly, however, there are several notable variants.

Hydrosalpinx, the "burned-out" remnants of a pyosalpinx can take two forms. The **simplex** form consists of a single thin-walled chamber with flattened mucosal folds. The **follicularis** form with many loculated compartments.

**Salpingitis isthmica nodosa** appears as gross nodulation of the isthmic portion of the fallopian tubes. The cross-sectional appearance is one of multiple small lumina. The risk of ectopic pregnancy is increased. This change adds mass to the tubes and can thus be mistaken for a cornual fibroid on vaginal examination. Chronic ovarian involvement can cause chronic perio-ophoritis.

*Clinical.* Clinical presentation is usually prompted by infertility or low-grade pelvic pain. Pelvic examination is often fruitless but detection of an adnexal mass suggesting abscess may be helpful. Diagnostic laparoscopy is often helpful.

*Treatment.* Antibiotic therapy is warranted if there is evidence of active infection. If pelvic pain persists despite antibiotics then extirpative surgery (TAH/BSO) is indicated provided the patient is no longer interested in retaining fertility. If, however, infertility is the reason for presentation then a variety of procedures (salpingolysis, salpingoplasty) are available but have limited success.

## Tubercular Salpingitis

Tubercular salpingitis is uncommon (< 5% incidence) in North America. It is important to consider the diagnosis because tubercular salpingitis usually responds to conservative therapy. Tuberculous salpingitis is the result of hematogenous dissemination from primary extragenital (usually pulmonary) sites of infection.

*Pathology.* Grossly the infection resembles that of the pyogenic salpingitis. Miliary dissemination with peritoneal seeding leads to a nodular exosalpingitis resembling salpingitis isthmica nodosa. Caseating granulomas are typically seen on microscopic examination.

Positive acid-fast bacilli (AFB) smears are suggestive and positive cultures are conclusive evidence of *M. tuberculosis* infection.

Tuberculous endometritis can result from contiguous spread and can be difficult to distinguish from endometrial adenocarcinoma microscopically. AFB studies are falsely negative in up to 50% of cases. Ovarian involvement (perio-ophoritis) is a rare complication. Vaginovulvar tuberculosis can present as a ragged ulcer resembling a treponemal chancre. Such lesions warrant biopsy to rule out malignancy.

*Clinical.* Tubercular salpingitis is difficult to distinguish clinically from other forms of chronic tubal infection. Circumstantial evidence includes a history of extragenital TB in the past, adnexal mass lesion in an individual having had no prior sexual intercourse, and salpingitis refractory to therapy that should be effective for the usual pathogens (Table 4-11).

*Treatment.* Standard antituberculous antibiotic therapy is indicated and may preserve reproductive capacity. Surgical excision may be necessary if conservative measures fail.

## Endometriosis

Endometriosis is defined as ectopic endometrial tissue. It can occur in many locations (listed in order of frequency): ovaries, pouch of Douglas, uterosacral ligaments, round ligament, fallopian tubes, and uterine serosa. Other less common sites include: uterine cervix, vagina, vermiform appendix, urinary bladder, and colon. Very rarely it is seen in laparotomy scars, the umbilicus, the lungs, and the kidneys. Endometrial tissue has been documented in the pelvic lymphatic channels and nodes suggesting that distant dissemination occurs through the lymphatics.

*Adenomyosis* is the name given to endometrial tissue within the uterine musculature. The term adenomyoma is used if the intramyometrial endometrium becomes circumscribed and nodular. Adenomyosis, if hormonally responsive, leads to the formation of intramural hematomas; adenomyoma is occasionally mistaken for a leiomyoma but it lacks the pseudocapsule characteristic of leiomyoma. Adenomyosis causes dysmenorrhea and menorrhagia similar to endometriosis, however, unlike endometriosis, ade-

Adenomyosis — endometrial tissue w/in the uterine musculature.

— lacks pseudocap char of biomyoma

nomyosis tends to occur in older (> 40 yr) parous women. Furthermore, adenomyosis can be difficult to distinguish pathologically from a well-differentiated endometrial adenocarcinoma. Endometriosis at the ovary can also lead to hematoma formation. The colloquial term *chocolate cyst* refers to the brown discoloration within an ovarian cyst due to retained hemosiderin.

*Clinical.* It is important to note that the degree of discomfort experienced-endometriosis bears no relationship to the amount of ectopic endometrium (see Table 4-10). Nonfunctional (i.e., sex steroid refractory) patches of ectopic endometrium do not cause symptoms. Infertility secondary to endometriosis is difficult to treat. Conventional hormonal therapy involves the use of synthetic progestins that are modified androgens or mild androgens that relieve symptoms but impair reproductive capacity during therapy by inducing amenorrhea.

*Pathogenesis.* There are three current theories regarding the formation of endometriosis lesions. The **transportation** concept (Samson's theory) proposes that there is a retrograde flow of menstrual fragments through the fallopian tubes onto the ovaries and the pelvic peritoneum. This might adequately explain lesions within proximity of the fallopian tubes but lymphatic and hematogenous dissemination have to be invoked for distant lesions. The theory of **formation-in-situ** invokes cellular metaplasia of the coelomic epithelium due to unexplained hormonal influences. The concept of **induction** represents a combination of the two postulates: refluxed menstrual fragments necrose but induce metaplasia in the adjacent coelomic epithelium. Currently the induction theory is most popular.

*Treatment.* The goals of therapy are: (1) to relieve pain and (2) to restore fertility. This can be accomplished by means of either hormonal therapy or surgery.

Generally hormonal therapy involves the use of progestins, mild synthetic androgens, or low-dose potent androgens and the avoidance of estrogens. Progestins, e.g., norethynodrel, in doses of up to 40 mg/day are used to induce a state of "pseudopregnancy." The regular withdrawal of

*norethynodrel   40 mg/day → pseudopregnancy*

Danazol - mild anti estrogenic + androgenic properties

progestational influence underlies regular endometrial shedding; conversely the persistent presence of progestin prevents endometrial sloughing. Furthermore the progestational predominance results in endometrial atrophy. Chronic progestin therapy also yields an endometrial surface highly unlikely to sustain nidation. Progestins are used for several months in an attempt to induce partial disease regression so that their discontinuation can be tolerated without recurrence of symptoms while restoring fertility.

Androgens have been noted to promote regression of endometriosis, whereas estrogens promote extension. Danazol (400–800 mg/d) is a synthetic steroid with mild antiestrogenic and androgenic properties that has been effective for pain relief and restoring fertility. Danazol may act by suppressing gonadotropin release from the pituitary, thus leading to a decline in ovarian estrogen production. The incidence of virilizing side effects is relatively low.

Surgical therapy is indicated for severe or hormone refractory disease. The goal is to rid the pelvis of as many endometriosis lesions as possible either by fulgeration or excision. If reproductive capacity need not be salvaged extirpative surgery can be performed. Total castration is not desirable in relatively young patients because of the potential complications of prolonged menopause, e.g., osteoporosis. The preservation of one adnexa is therefore usually advisable.

## Ectopic Pregnancy

Defined as implantation of the conceptus anywhere other than the endometrial cavity. Most ectopics (>95%) occur in the fallopian tubes. The majority of these occur in the ampullary portion of the tube. Ectopic pregnancy is the leading cause of maternal mortality in the first trimester. The major clinical problems with ectopics are circulatory collapse (exsanguination) and subsequent compromise of fertility.

*Etiology.* The etiology is multifactorial. Several factors that have been implicated include: (1) rising incidence of salpingitis and (2) rising incidence of tubal surgery. The association with certain other factors is still controversial including: IUDs, abortion, progestin-only OCPs, and postcoital estrogens for abortion.

majority of ectopics occur in ampullary portion of tube.

Sexual promiscuity increases the risk of exposure to venereal pathogens and salpingitis. Aggressive antibiotic therapy for salpingitis may be preserving tubal patency but does not prevent intratubal damage altogether thereby perhaps increasing the risk of tubal nidation. There is a higher prevalence of salpingitis isthmica nodosa in populations where tubal pregnancy is more common (West Indies).

There is a higher prevalence of tubal surgery (e.g., tubal ligation, salpingoplasty) in patients with ectopics. Tubal ligation by cautery is the method most often associated with subsequent ectopics. In general the risk for tubal implantation is greatest during the first 3 postoperative years.

Intrauterine devices, abortion, and the progestin-only OCPs are believed to increase the risk of subsequent tubal implantation. These agents selectively diminish the suitability of the uterine cavity to nidation. Progestin-laden IUDs may be more hazardous than others. Tubal surgery and postcoital estrogen preparations promote tubal implantation perhaps by means of altered tubal function. (↑ esTrogens caused cilia dysfunction)

**Pathogenesis.** After the conceptus implants ectopically the chorionic villi begin eroding into the underlying tissues. The tubal wall is not thick enough to sustain this process, thus the conceptus ruptures the tube and any vascular channels in its path.

**Clinical.** The classic triad is that of: (1) pain, (2) vaginal bleeding, and (3) adnexal mass (see Table 4-10). The vaginal hemorrhage is usually minimal in comparison with that which accompanies spontaneous (incomplete) abortion. Vaginal hemorrhage occurs when the progestational support of the conceptus for the endometrial surface fails.

**Diagnostic Considerations.** The most useful investigations are: (1) β-HCG radioimmunoassay and (2) pelvic ultrasound (U/S). Culdocentesis may also be helpful.

Ultrasound is used to detect an intrauterine gestational sac and rule out the diagnosis of ectopic pregnancy. Only very rarely are intrauterine and ectopic pregnancy coexistent (1/30,000). The absence of an intrauterine gestational sac with a positive βHCG is consistent with diagnosis of ectopic

*- T₁/₂ βhCG = 12 hrs*

*- Defibrinated blood in Cul de Sac*

pregnancy in ~50% of cases. The detection of an adnexal mass is too nonspecific to permit the diagnosis of a tubal pregnancy. A fetal heart detected within an adnexal (or extrauterine) mass is a rare (5%) but definitive finding of ectopic gestation.

A brief review of human chorionic gonadotropin (HCG) kinetics is in order at this point. During early, normal intrauterine pregnancy the HCG level doubles every day or two (100% increase q24–48 h). HCG begins to decline as soon as pregnancy is terminated with a half-life of approximately 12 hours (levels decline to ~4% of initial value within 72 hours). A single beta-HCG value is not as helpful as serial determinations. Either an insufficiently rapid rise (< 66% increase in 48 hours) or a decline of any magnitude in the beta-HCG level is consistent with a diagnosis of ectopic pregnancy.

Culdocentesis is performed to document the presence of defibrinated blood consistent with hemoperitoneum. This requires tubal rupture to have already occurred. A false-negative result (no blood aspirated) may be encountered if the cul-de-sac is obliterated by prior inflammatory disease or endometriosis lesions.

Laparoscopy provides direct visualization of the tubes but they must be viewed in their entirety, from fimbria to uterus, to accurately rule out the diagnosis.

**Treatment.** The list of possible surgical procedures has lengthened recently with a definite trend toward a more conservative approach aimed at optimizing subsequent reproductive capacity. Possible procedures include: salpingectomy, salpingo-oopherectomy, linear salpingostomy (laparoscopic/laparotomy), segmental resection with or without reanastomosis (laparoscopic/laparotomy), or tubal "milking" at laparotomy. Salpingectomy is still the most common procedure.

Linear salpingostomy is suggested for hemodynamically stable patients with unruptured ampullary implantation of less than 3 cm dilatation. Segmental resection is thought to be particularly amenable to the uniform-calibre isthmic implantations that are freely mobile and less than 3 cm dilated.

*⚹ Medical Tx: methotrexate Rx*

**Prognosis.** Subsequent fertility is relatively poor with 25% to 45% term pregnancy rates and 10% to 20% subsequent recurrence rate of tubal nida-

*Procidentia = gross external prolapse of uterus.*

tion. Conservative surgery improves postoperative patency rates but may not increase fertility significantly.

## UTEROVAGINAL PROLAPSE

Prolapse is defined as the downward displacement of a part or viscus. In this section the prolapse of the pelvic organs into the vagina is reviewed. This topic goes by many other names: genital prolapse, pelvic floor relaxation, or simply vaginal relaxation. The pathophysiology of the process is not complicated: trauma or an inherent weakness (or most commonly a combination of the two) of the structures that support the pelvic organs can eventually result in their failure to maintain these organs in their proper positions and they descend.

*Etiology.* The most common form of pelvic trauma is normal childbirth. Weakness of the pelvic support ligaments may be congenital (rare) or due to postmenopausal atrophy (common). Trauma by itself, in an otherwise healthy young woman, is rarely sufficient to cause prolapse. The additive effect of postmenopausal atrophy is responsible for clinical presentation and therefore the high incidence in this age group. Disorders that chronically raise intra-abdominal pressure (COPD, obesity) also play a contributory role.

*Classification.* Simple anatomic classification refers to the vaginal wall through which the offending organ transgresses.

| Anterior Segment | Superior Segment | Posterior Segment |
|---|---|---|
| Urethrocoele | Uterine | Rectocoele |
| Cystocoele | Vaginal vault | Enterocoele |

"Coele" is the suffix that designates prolapse, the prefix gives the organ involved. Cystocoele refers to prolapse of the urinary bladder. Urethrocoele is prolapse of the urethra. The vaginal vault may descend after hysterectomy resembling intussusception. Uterine prolapse is subdivided into partial descent (cervix proximal to introitus), descent of the cervix to the vestibule, and finally gross external prolapse or procidentia. Enterocoele

*True hernia*

refers to the distal small bowel prolapsing through the uterorectal pouch (pouch of Douglas); rectocoeles occur at the same location.

***Clinical.*** Patients may complain of a vague heavy sensation, "a lump coming down," or a feeling of pressure in the pelvis. Backache that sometimes also occurs is due to secondary postural adjustments.

With urethrocoele or cystocoele there may also be bladder irritability symptoms (frequency, urgency, dysuria) as well as stress incontinence (involuntary escape of urine accompanying transient elevations in intrapelvic pressure) with coughing and sneezing. Cystocoele can lead to cystitis and possibly pyelonephritis by promoting urinary stasis. Tenesmus is often noted with rectocoeles and the patient may give a history of the need for transvaginal digital reduction to permit complete defecation.

***Anatomy Review.*** The prerequisite pathophysiologic event is the weakening of the endopelvic fascia that lies between the levatores ani muscle sheath and the urogenital diaphragm. Synonymous expressions for endopelvic fascia include parametrium and visceral pelvic fascia.

This fascia can be subdivided according to the type of organ it invests and supports. There are **visceral sheaths** that invest the bladder, the rectum, and the vagina. The latter being particularly strong. **Muscle sheaths** envelope the levatores ani and the sphincter urethrae together with the deep transverse perineal muscles. The **paracervical fascia** or false parametrial ligaments represent condensations of the endopelvic fascia into three pairs of cervical supporting structures: pubocervical, uterosacral, and transverse cervical (cardinal or Mackenrodt) ligaments. The pubocervical ligaments are actually made up of the pubovesical and vesicocervical components. Of the paracervical fascia the transverse ligaments are chief in the prevention of cervical prolapse, whereas the uterosacrals are most important in preventing posterior segment prolapse.

***Treatment.*** The most effective form of therapy is surgical repair, however, should the patient not be a surgical candidate pessaries become a reasonable alternative. Topical estrogen preparations are usually combined with pessaries to strengthen the vaginal epithelium and prevent mechanical ulceration.

*Cardinal ligaments prevent cervical prolapse*
*Uterosacrals prevent posterior segment prolapse*

As the weak fascia gives way and prolapses, it stretches the preceding epithelium. Surgical correction addresses these two problems through resection of the redundant epithelium and reinforcement of the underlying fascia with strong nonreabsorbable suture material. For both superior and upper posterior prolapse, hysterectomy facilitates resuspension of the lagging structure by permitting use of the freed parametrial ligaments.

## BREAST CARCINOMA SCREENING

### Breast Lump Evaluation

Breast carcinoma is the most common site of cancer (27%) and the most common cause of cancer-related death (19%) in women. The incidence of breast cancer in the general female population is 6%. The incidence peaks in the 50- to 55-year age group. Early detection through screening studies can diminish morbidity and mortality. Efficacious screening tests must have high sensitivities so that the number of false-negative results will be negligible. High specificity, although desirable is less important.

Of the currently available techniques for breast carcinoma screening only two, breast self-examination and mammography, have gained universal approval. The former involves regular monthly systematic palpation of both breasts by the female population at large (> 35 years of age). The latter is a technically modified form of radiography that enhances resolution within soft tissues. There are in fact two forms of mammography currently available, **screen-film** and **xeroradiography.** The former requires a dedicated machine but delivers a slightly lower dose of radiation per exposure (0.2 rad vs. 0.4 rad). The overall accuracy of lesion detection and the extrapolated risk of inducing carcinoma (estimated at 1 excess case of malignancy per 1,000,000 women examined) are not technique dependent.

Breast screening studies identify lesions with the following degree of reliability (Table 4-12).

Note that palpable lesions have a 20% specificity for malignancy, whereas mammographically detected lesions have a 10% specificity for malignancy.

Methods currently available for the investigation of breast lumps fall into two groups: those that distinguish benign from malignant lesions (physi-

$$\text{Sensitivity} = \frac{TP}{TP + FN}$$

**TABLE 4-12. MALIGNANCY DETECTION IN BREAST SCREENING STUDIES**

| Method | Malignancy Detection | |
| --- | --- | --- |
| | *Sensitivity* | *Specificity* |
| Breast self-examination | 35% | |
| Mammography | 75% | 90% |

cian breast examination, mammography, cytologic or histologic examination) and those that distinguish adjunctive traits (ultrasound).

Clinical traits that increase the risk of malignancy include: a positive family (first degree relatives) history of breast cancer, past history of breast cancer, and advancing age. Nipple secretion is nonspecific, indeed a bloody secretion is suggestive of intraductal papilloma (benign lesion) and serous secretions can occur in patients taking antidopaminergic agents.

It is conventionally assumed that 90% of benign breast lumps are soft/cystic, mobile, and possess a regular margin, therefore, the following reliability can be ascribed to these signs (Table 4-13).

Obvious skin retraction, nipple inversion, or peau d'orange appearance of the skin overlying the breast are highly suggestive of malignancy. The same is true of palpable axillary or supraclavicular lymph nodes in the absence of regional infection.

Mammographic traits characteristic of malignancy have been defined, therefore mammography can be used to diagnose malignancy of breast lesions as well as simple detection of breast lesions. Mammography, when

**TABLE 4-13. ACCURACY OF PHYSICAL FINDINGS SUGGESTIVE OF MALIGNANCY IN BREAST MASSES**

| Sign | Malignancy Detection | |
| --- | --- | --- |
| | *Sensitivity* | *Specificity* |
| Irregular margin | 60% | 90% |
| (Not soft/cystic) Firm | 60% | 90% |
| (Not mobile) Fixed | 40% | 90% |

used to distinguish between malignant and benign breast lesions, has a sensitivity of 85% and a specificity of 95%. Thus a mammographically malignant lesion should be resected and a mammographically benign lesion can confidently be followed without surgical intervention.

Breast ultrasonography can be used to distinguish malignant from benign breast lesions or to distinguish cystic lesions from solid ones. In the former capacity the sensitivity and specificity of breast ultrasonography are worse than for mammography. In the latter capacity this procedure can be very helpful (sensitivity and specificity ~99.9%). If a lesion is clinically suspect as being cystic and sonography documents this fact, then fine-needle aspiration and cytologic examination of its contents can be attempted. This spares the patient mammography and potentially biopsy.

Fine-needle aspiration is a relatively simple office procedure. The complication rate is low and the procedure yields material adequate for cytologic examination ~95% of the time (for masses > 0.5 cm diameter). Cytology for the detection of malignancy has a sensitivity of 95% and a specificity of 98%. Furthermore if the results indicate a benign lesion, and aspiration has been complete, a cure has been effected.

A suggested approach for breast lesion detection and breast lesion evaluation is given in Figure 4-3.

# CARCINOMA OF THE CERVIX

The incidence of squamous cell carcinoma of the cervix, once the most common malignancy of the female reproductive tract, has recently begun to decline primarily as the result of vigorous screening programs. There is circumstantial evidence relating cervical neoplasia to ethnic background (decreased incidence for the Jewish population), racial factors (increased incidence in blacks and Puerto Ricans), sexual habit (increased incidence in women who initiated sexual activity when < 20 years old and have multiple partners), and with certain infections, notably $HSV_2$. The true etiology of the disorder is not known.

**Pathology.** Microscopically the majority of cervical carcinoma lesions reveal squamous cell histology (90%), the remainder are adenocarcinomas

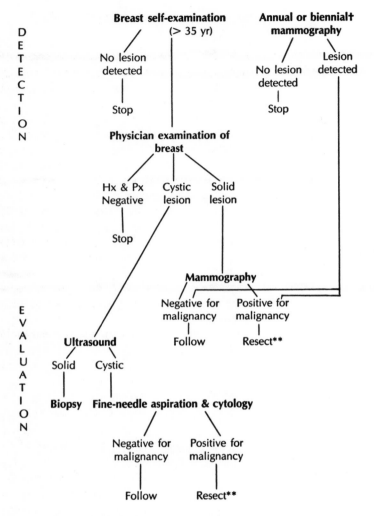

D
E
T
E
C
T
I
O
N

E
V
A
L
U
A
T
I
O
N

**Breast self-examination**
(> 35 yr)

No lesion
detected

Stop

**Annual or biennial†**
**mammography**

No lesion
detected

Lesion
detected

Stop

**Physician examination of**
**breast**

Hx & Px        Cystic      Solid
Negative       lesion      lesion

Stop

**Mammography**

Negative for        Positive for
malignancy          malignancy

Follow              Resect**

**Ultrasound**

Solid       Cystic

**Biopsy   Fine-needle aspiration & cytology**

Negative for        Positive for
malignancy          malignancy

Follow              Resect**

**, increasingly the trend is toward more conservative primary resections supplemented with radiotherapy. †, American College of Physicians recommends screening mammography between 50–59 years of age (this is controversial).

**Figure 4-3.** Breast lesion detection & evaluation.

142

exophytic : endophytic
      2            1

(originating within the endocervical canal) adenosquamous carcinomas, sarcomas, and melanomas. Adenosquamous lesions possess both glandular and squamous epithelial components and have the worst prognosis. The prognosis for adenocarcinomas falls somewhere between that of squamous cell and adenosquamous cell lesions.

Macroscopically, carcinoma-in-situ (CIS) and cervical intraepithelial neoplasia (CIN) are clinically indistinguishable from the surrounding normal epithelium. Early invasive disease presents as a small, firm mass at or near the external cervical os with a granular and friable surface that may bleed on contact. The lesion may be difficult to identify and distinguish from surrounding chronic inflammatory changes or from physiologic eversion.

Moderately advanced lesions are more often exophytic (growing above the surface) than endophytic (growing beneath the surface) in a ratio of almost 2:1. Far advanced disease results in gross destruction of the cervix with ulceration, leaving a very friable surface. Adjacent vaginal walls are often hardened with infiltrating tumor. When the broad ligament becomes involved the ureters may become occluded causing obstructive renal failure. Involvement of the bladder and bowels can lead to fistulization.

Lymphatic metastases reach the iliac, para-aortic, and then more distant nodes. Common sites of distant visceral metastases include lungs, liver, bone, and brain. Death most commonly results from local infiltration (ureteric obstruction) leading to renal failure. The next most common causes of death are sepsis and hemorrhage.

① Renal Failure
② sepsis / hemorrhage

*Pathogenesis.* The most constant fact about cervical carcinoma is that it tends to arise at the squamocolumnar junction otherwise known as the transformation or T zone. Physiologic cervical *eversion* is the exposure of endocervical mucous-secreting columnar epithelium to the vaginal canal. Eversion occurs at menarch or with first pregnancy. Eversion can be confused with carcinoma on first inspection.

Adenocarcinoma originates in the cervical canal and has a distinctive atypical gland pattern on histologic examination. Detection of a glandular component within tumour biopsy mandates the performance of a fractional dilatation and curettage (D & C) to ascertain whether the uterine corpus is involved.

*Classification.* Dysplasia is the reversible partial dedifferentiation of mature tissue (in this case epithelium); CIS is the full thickness replacement of an epithelium by malignant appearing cells **without** penetration of the underlying basement membrane. The degree of dysplasia can then be divided into mild, moderate, and severe according to the depth of the epithelium that is involved, i.e., mild, only the lower one third; moderate, the lower two thirds; and severe, the upper one third is also involved but not completely. This classification then has five gradations from mild dysplasia through moderate and severe dysplasia to CIS and finally to frank malignancy. The only distinction between CIS but not frank malignancy is the penetration of the basement membrane by malignant cells in the latter.

The newer classification system has four gradations beginning with CIN-1 (cervical intraepithelial neoplasia), roughly equivalent to mild dysplasia; CIN-2 similar to moderate dysplasia; CIN-3, which includes both severe dysplasia and CIS and frank malignancy.

The average age of occurrence of dysplasia is 32 years, 38 years for CIS, and 48 years for carcinoma. Dysplastic epithelium almost always demonstrates an acquired chromosomal aneuploidy that may become a helpful tool in distinguishing such cells from their normal counterparts if no other method succeeds. The histologic classifications delineated have little prognostic value beyond defining the presence or absence of basement membrane penetration.

*Clinical Presentation.* Unfortunately intraepithelial disease is most often asymptomatic, whereas invasive disease usually presents as posttraumatic (either postcoital or after straining at stool) vaginal bleeding. If the lesion is primarily endocervical then it may be clinically silent for a longer period. Adenocarcinomas present with pink or blood-tinged vaginal discharge that subsequently proceeds to frank bleeding. As the disease progresses the discharge may become foul smelling due to infection. When the vesicovaginal septum becomes involved symptoms of bladder irritation, (urgency, frequency, and nocturia) may appear. Rectal discomfort or pain suggests posterior extension of the lesion. The triad of persistent lumbosacral pain, unilateral lymphedema, and unilateral ureteric obstruction is usually associated with an incurable degree of extension.

***Diagnostic Studies.*** The *Papanicolaou* (PAP) *smear* (exfoliative cytologic method) is a reasonably good screening procedure but does not localize lesions and it has a false-negative rate of up to 20%. The physician collecting the sample must indicate when the smear is taken (with respect to the patient's menstrual cycle) to permit accurate cytologic interpretation.

The *Schiller test* refers to the application of either Schiller's 0.3% or Lugol's 5.0% iodine solution to the cervix. Normal squamous cells are stained a mahogany brown color, whereas rapidly dividing, dysplastic cells remain unstained due to their lack of glycogen, unfortunately normal columnar epithelium also fails to be stained therefore Schiller positive (unstained) regions near the squamocolumnar junction may be endocervical epithelium or dysplastic cells.

*Colposcopy* (discussed further in a separate section) is used to localize lesions detected by cytologic methods for effective biopsy. Colposcopy is now widely used to follow up on abnormal Pap smears and to permit accurate directed cervical biopsies.

*Cone biopsy* refers to excision of the cervix and a portion of the distal endocervical canal and contains the entire squamocolumnar junction. It is indicated when: (1) colposcopic examination is unsatisfactory (squamocolumnar junction not visualized); (2) the lesion extends into the cervical canal; or when (3) the cytologic and colposcopic findings do not match. Cone biopsy is being performed less often now that colposcopy is proving to be quite useful. The chief complications are hemorrhage and cervical incompetence.

***Clinical Staging.*** The clinical staging system rather than the histologic classification bears both prognostic and therapeutic significance (Table 4-14).

***Treatment.*** The most effective treatment for stage 0 disease is simple, vaginal or abdominal, hysterectomy with ovarian conservation. For the patient who wishes to retain reproductive capacity either laser, cautery, cryotherapy, or conization is indicated. None of these latter methods is totally successful, conization has a 9% failure rate, other methods may have even worse failure rates. Failures are more common when undetected endo-

Conization Complications (9% Failure Rate)
① hemorrhage
② cervical incompetence.

*Invasive disease insensitive to Chemotx agents,*

**TABLE 4-14. CLINICAL STAGING FOR CARCINOMA OF THE CERVIX**

| | |
|---|---|
| Stage 0 | Carcinoma-in-situ (CIS) |
| Stage 1 | Cervix only, involved |
| | (a) Microinvasive disease (< 5 mm) *depth* |
| | (b) Other than microinvasive  $|a_2)$ *horizontal 7mm* |
| Stage 2 | (a) Upper two thirds of vagina involved |
| | (b) Parametrial involvement *(Ligaments)* |
| Stage 3 | (a) Lower one third of vagina involved |
| | (b) Pelvic side-wall involved |
| Stage 4 | (a) Adjacent pelvic organ involvement |
| | (b) Distant visceral metastases |

cervical extension is present. Those women who choose therapy other than simple hysterectomy must be followed closely.

To make the diagnosis of microinvasive disease one must visualize the entire region by means of a cone biopsy. Microinvasive disease is defined as < 3 mm penetration of the basement membrane without lymphatic invasion or confluence in the pattern of invasion. Simple hysterectomy is usually sufficient. If, however, the depth of invasion is between 3 and 5 mm or the lymphatics are involved a radical (Wertheim) hysterectomy is available.

Invasive disease is insensitive to the chemotherapeutic agents currently available. Radiotherapy can take the form of external radiation when there is a large tumor with paracervical and pelvic lymph node spread or intracavitary radiation for small tumors or postoperative remnants following surgical debulking. Minor radiation side effects include: bladder irritability, diarrhea, skin changes, and transient rectal bleeding. A major complication is fistulization to the bladder or the rectum. Radiated tissues are replaced by fragile, hypovascular tissues that breakdown readily to form fistulae. Surgery within irradiated fields is more often complicated by poor wound healing and dehiscence.

Radical hysterectomy with pelvic node dissection may be indicated for stage 1(b) or stage 2(a) disease provided the patient is medically fit for surgery (~75%). If surgery is inadvisable, then radiotherapy is suggested.

Cervical carcinoma is uncommon during pregnancy (0.005%). Intraepithelial disease can be treated conservatively with conization and the pregnancy carried to term. Invasive disease presenting before 26 weeks' gestation, may warrant termination of the pregnancy and institution of regular treatment. If invasive disease discovered after the 26th week then a cesarean section may be performed at 34 to 36 weeks LMP and treatment instituted as usual. The survival rates are the same as for nonpregnant patients using this approach. Pregnancy has no effect on the staging or progression of cervical carcinoma.

Follow-up consists of vaginal examination, Pap smear and palpation of the regional and supraclavicular nodes. Initially every 3 months for 1 year, then every 4 months for another year, and finally every 6 months for the next 3 years. Central pelvic or vaginal vault recurrences are curable and thus warrant full workup. Anterior pelvic exenteration with ileal conduit or posterior pelvic exenteration with colostomy (whichever will best address the site of recurrence) may be indicated. Total pelvic exenteration may be beneficial for selected patients.

## COLPOSCOPY

Colposcopy is a technique by which the uterine cervix can be visualized under a bright light at magnifications of 6× to 40×. Such visualization is intended to permit: (1) determination of the degree of dysplasia and (2) directed or localized biopsy as opposed to a blind or a random choice biopsy site.

The premise upon which colposcopy rests is that progressive characteristic changes occur in the vasculature and superficial cells of the cervix as it becomes more dysplastic. Pap smear & colposcopy have been shown to be complimentary in carcinoma detection.

The cervix is examined through the colposcope both before and after the application of acetic acid. Increasing degrees of dysplasia are characterized by: (1) increased intercapillary distance, (2) elevation of the surface, and (3) color change from pink to white upon application of acetic acid (Table 4-15).

In review, the three major diagnostic modalities for determining the

**TABLE 4-15. COLPOSCOPIC TERMINOLOGY**

| Terminology | Description | Acetic Acid |
|---|---|---|
| Unsatisfactory examination | Squamocolumnar junction not visualized | |
| **Normal Tissue** | | |
| Original squamous epithelium | Nonspecific appearance | Pink |
| Columnar epithelium | Nonspecific appearance | Grapelike |
| Transformation zone (T zone) | Nonspecific appearance | Tongues of grapes. |
| **Dysplasia to CIS** | | |
| White epithelium | A well-demarcated region that changes color in response to Acetic Acid | White |
| Punctate epithelium | Stippled vessels; well demarcated | White |
| Mosaic epithelium | Mosaic vessels; well demarcated | White |
| **CIS to Carcinoma** | | |
| Leukoplakia | Well-demarcated region that appears white before the application of $CH_3COOH$ | N/A |
| Atypical vessels | Bizarre appearing vessels, some parallel to surface | N/A |

*Note:* Normal tissues are pink both before and after the application of acetic acid; leukoplakia used in this context is a specific colposcopic term defined in Table.

presence of cervical carcinoma are: (1) biopsy with definitive histologic examination, (2) cytology in the form of a Pap smear, and (3) colposcopy. The first, although definitive, is time-consuming and costly; cytology is a good screening test but has a significant number of false-negative results; colposcopy has less false-negative results but does not always visualize the endocervix. Cone biopsy is the most sensitive procedure because one visualizes the entire squamocolumnar junction and cervical canal. This procedure, however, requires hospital admission and may promote cervical incompetence and therefore spontaneous midtrimester abortion.

Figure 4-4 is a composite approach to the diagnosis of cervical carcinoma.

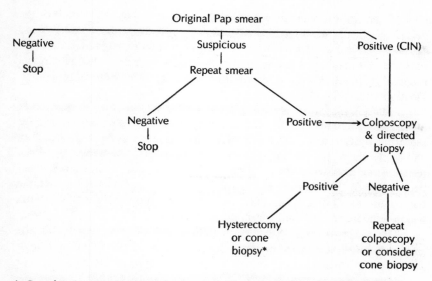

*, Cone biopsy may represent adequate surgical excision for those patients who wish to preserve fertility. *Note:* The endocervical canal must be visualized either by colposcopy or histologically for staging purposes.

**Figure 4-4.** Composite approach to the diagnosis of cervical carcinoma.

## LEIOMYOMA    *Most common tumor of uterus.*

Leiomyoma also known as fibroid or simply myoma is a benign neoplasm of uterine smooth muscle. It is the most common tumor of the uterus. Up to 20% of women in the general population have fibroids (higher incidence among blacks). Fibroids occur almost exclusively during childbearing years, they rarely develop de novo postmenopausally, and in fact they usually tend to regress postmenopausally. Postmenopausal increase in size of a fibroid is rare but is highly suggestive of sarcomatous (malignant) transformation.

*most common to → submucosal = 5%*
*get infected*

*subserosal → do not cause DUB*

*intramural → most common*

*but can cause ureteric obstruction*

**Classification.** Myomas may involve the uterine corpus (corporeal) or the cervix (cervical). Corporeal myomas are much more common than cervical lesions. Cervical myomas can cause GU obstruction through urethral compression and may become impacted within the bony pelvis making surgical removal difficult. Corporeal fibroids are best classified according to their location within the uterine wall.

Approximately 5% are located just beneath the endometrial surface, submucosal. Submucosal myomas are the most likely to cause hemorrhage requiring hysterectomy. The overlying mucosa tends to be thin, atrophic, and easily ulcerated. For unknown reasons they are also at increased risk for sarcomatous transformation. Submucosal lesions, can be either sessile or pedunculated. The former are at times detected as "bumps" under the curette during D & C. The latter may protrude from the cervical os and become ulcerated, infected, or strangulated.

The most common variety of myoma is located entirely within the myometrium, intramural or interstitial. Large or multiple intramural myomas can cause marked uterine enlargement with dysmenorrhea.

Myomas may also be located just beneath the uterine serosa, subserosal. Pedunculated subserosal fibroids have the unique capability of eventually deriving this blood supply from the parietal peritoneum rather than from the uterine corpus. Such lesions are referred to as "parasitic" myomas. Subserosal fibroids can cause ureteric obstruction as well as iliac vascular occlusion. The superficial venous passages of these lesions can, if they rupture, cause massive intraperitoneal hemorrhage.

There exist three rare variant forms of fibroids that are mentioned here only briefly. **Intravenous leiomyomatosis** refers to the direct extension of a lesion into the veins adjacent to the uterus. Histologically benign, this form of fibroid can result in fatal pulmonary embolization. **Leiomyomatosis peritonealis disseminata** is a very rare form of the disease almost always seen during pregnancy or the puerperium and consists of multiple subparietal–peritoneal lesions. It is also histologically benign and does not lead to distant metastases. **Benign metastatic** myoma refers to distant metastases (e.g., lung) with the microscopic appearance of a myoma. The choice of name is unfortunate because this is considered a low-grade form of sarcoma.

**Pathology.** Microscopically myomas appear as interlacing whorls of spin-

*mildly estrogen dependent*

dle-shaped smooth muscle cells with a variable component of connective tissue. There is no true capsule but surgery is facilitated by a pseudocapsule formed by the compressed, adjacent nonneoplastic myometrium. The gross pathology is described within the classification.

*Secondary Changes.* Secondary or degenerative changes of fibroids are very characteristic of this entity and are often solely responsible for clinical presentation (Table 4-16).

*Etiology.* The etiology is unknown. Myomas are mildly estrogen-dependent as evidenced by their tendency to (1) appear during childbearing years, (2) grow during pregnancy, and (3) regress postmenopausally.

*Signs and Symptoms.* Most often myomas are asymptomatic incidental findings on physical examination. They present as either abdominal or adnexal masses on abdominal or vaginal examination, respectively. Alter-

**TABLE 4-16. DEGENERATIVE CHANGES OF FIBROIDS**

| Degeneration Type | Description |
| --- | --- |
| Hyaline | The most common form of degeneration; seen to some extent in all fibroids. Cytoplasm takes on a glossy homogeneous appearance |
| Cystic | After hyalinization fibroids tend to liquifaction becoming large cystic cavities. They can be mistaken for pregnancy, ovarian cyst, or lymphangioma (if lymphatic blockage and lymphedema occur) |
| Calcification | More likely if there is impairment of the vascular supply. Form fruste = "wombstone" |
| Infection | Most likely with submucous fibroids with thin overlying protective endometrial tissue |
| Necrosis | Secondary to infection, infarction, or torsion |
| Carnerous ("red") | Rare; usually during pregnancy. May represent asceptic necrosis with hemolysis |
| Fatty | Rare; after advanced hyalinization |
| Sarcomatous | Extremely rare; malignant transformation |

natively they can present with hypermenorrhea, pain, or pressure effects on the surrounding pelvic viscera.

On abdominal examination a firm, irregular, nodular, nontender, and often mobile mass in a woman of childbearing age is consistent with the diagnosis of leiomyoma. Nodular uterine masses found on digital pelvic examination may represent subserous fibroids, an abnormally flexed uterus, or an early pregnancy in an otherwise grossly myomatous uterus. Pedunculated subserous lesions must be distinguished from solid ovarian neoplasia. Submucous fibroids can be quite large without altering the size of the uterus, and therefore frequently escape diagnosis until hysterosalpingography or D & C is performed for other reasons.

Hypermenorrhea is the most common presenting complaint with fibroids. Both submucous or intramural lesions are capable of increasing endometrial surface area thereby increasing menstrual blood loss. Submucous myomas tend to cause more severe bleeding. Although fibroids can cause metrorrhagia, it is hazardous to assume a diagnosis of myoma in a metrorrhagic patient without ruling out carcinoma of the cervix and adenocarcinoma of the uterus. Subserous fibroids do not cause dysfunctional uterine bleeding (DUB).

Pain is a relatively unusual presenting complaint for uncomplicated myomas. The archtypical pain is usually described as a heavy sensation, with or without, dysmenorrhea. Pain and tenderness together with other signs of abdominal catastrophe in a patient with a previously asymptomatic fibroid are suggestive of torsion of a pedunculated myoma or some form of inflammatory degenerative change. Radicular pain may result from a large fibroid compressing the sacral plexus.

Large myomas can compress adjacent viscera. Bladder compression can cause dysuria, frequency, and urgency; ureteric compression can lead to hydronephrosis with secondary infection; bowel involvement may lead to subacute obstruction and rarely pelvic vein thrombosis due to venous obstruction.

*Complications*

## Pregnancy and Leiomyomas

Myoma, as a cause of infertility, can only be proposed when all other possibilities have been ruled out. Their size, number, and location relative to the cornua are variables that will govern whether they impede fertilization or

*↑ risk of uterine rupture during labor following myomectomy.*

nidation of the fertilized ovum. Those with fibroids judged to be the cause of infertility are candidates for myomectomy, but one must keep in mind that the uterine wall will be weakened with an increased risk of uterine rupture ✱ during labor.

Problems that can arise as a result of fibroids once pregnancy is ✱ achieved can be broken down by trimesters. Spontaneous first trimester abortion is the most common mode of pregnancy loss. The strategically placed lesion is a mechanical impediment to nidation. Red degeneration tends to occur during the second trimester with pain, fever, tenderness, and leukocytosis. This condition is managed conservatively with bedrest and analgesics. Should the situation become intolerable, induced abortion should be considered. C-section and hysterectomy may be advisable if pregnancy does proceed successfully because of the increased risk of uterine rupture associated with red degeneration. Third trimester problems center around labor. The fibroid acts as an impediment to effective forceful contraction, thus prolonging labor and leading to uterine atony, one of the major causes of peripartum hemorrhage. Initial clinical presentation of myoma during pregnancy is relatively common.

***Therapeutic Principles.*** An asymptomatic fibroid can be reevaluated every 6 months. If there is no change throughout the childbearing years, spontaneous postmenopausal regression should be awaited. Indications for resection, myomectomy, or hysterectomy include rapid enlargement or a myoma ✱ larger than a 12 week pregnant uterus. If myomectomy is planned, a D & C should precede the major procedure to rule out sinister occult lesions. Postmenopausal enlargement of a pelvic mass assumed to have been a ✓ myoma suggests either misdiagnosis of an ovarian neoplasm or sarcomatous degeneration. In either instance surgery is the intervention of choice.

*hys if myoma > 12 wk uterus*

## ENDOMETRIAL HYPERPLASIA AND POLYPS

In this section the normal cyclic variation in endometrial appearance is reviewed as is the appearance of hyperplastic endometrial proliferation and endometrial polyps.

*initial presentation of myoma during pregnancy is relatively common.*

*Basalis – progesterone refractory*

## Normal Endometrial Cycling

The endometrium is divided into three strata vertically from surface to myometrium: compact, spongy, and basalis layers. The compact and spongy layers are sloughed with every menstrual period (~q28d), whereas the basalis is the progesterone refractory layer responsible for endometrial regeneration.

By convention the 28-day cycle is taken as standard with day 1 defined as the first day of menstrual bleeding. During the initial 4 to 5 days of the cycle the microscopic appearance of the endometrium is one of superficial desquamation. The subsequent 4- to 5-day postmenstrual interval reveals a 1- to 2-mm thick endometrium with cuboidal surface epithelium, straight narrow glands, and dense compact stroma. The remainder of the *proliferative* (follicular, estrogenic, or preovulatory) portion of the cycle is typified by tall ciliated columnar surface epithelium with numerous mitotic figures visible.

After the midcycle luteinizing hormone (LH) surge triggers ovulation, the *secretory* (luteal, progestigenic, or postovulatory) portion of the menstrual cycle commences. The initial sign of secretory activity is the presence of subnuclear vacuoles in the epithelial cells. Glycogen granules can also be detected at this time, both intracellular and with glandlumina. The stroma becomes more vascular and more dense. The final days of this half of the cycle (premenstrual interval) are typified by a 5- to 7-mm thick endometrium with tall surface epithelium (as described earlier) but the glandular epithelial cells are short with frayed luminal edges and basal nuclei. The glandular architecture remains unchanged in the deeper basalis and compact layers, but in the spongy layer it becomes very tortuous with the glands taking on a corkscrew appearance. Stromal cells hypertrophy and become very loosely arranged, appearing edematous. Shortly thereafter the superficial layers are again sloughed and the cycle is renewed.

## Endometrial Hyperplasia

Hyperplasia, the abnormal increase in the number of normal cells in normal arrangement in a given tissue can arise anywhere in the body. The added interest in atypical adenomatous hyperplasia of the endometrium is sparked by the strong possibility that it represents a reversible premalignant change.

Androstenedione → estrone
Testosterone → estradiol

Hyperplasia of the endometrium is also a common cause of DUB, usually in the postmenopausal age group.

The hormone that causes endometrial proliferation is estrogen, thus any situation that results in continuous unopposed estrogen stimulation of the endometrium can lead to endometrial hyperplasia. The excess estrogenic stimulation can be exogenous or endogenous. Presently the vogue is to place postmenopausal women on estrogen supplements to prevent an as yet undefined subpopulation of such women from developing osteoporosis. If this supplementation is not cycled with a progestin to promote regular sloughing of the endometrium (mimicking regular menses), cystic hyperplasia may result.

Endogenous estrogen excess may arise directly from the ovaries as with polycystic ovarian disease (Stein-Levinthal syndrome), where multiple follicle cysts persistently generate estrogens. The follicles do not ovulate and thus do not progress to luteal structures that produce progestins that would result in sloughing upon withdrawal. A rare ovarian source of excess unopposed estrogen, granulosa cell tumor, is usually associated with precocious puberty. Obesity is also associated with estrogenic excess. Peripheral adipose tissue has the ability to convert androstenedione and testosterone to estrone ($E_1$) and estradiol ($E_2$), respectively. The androstenedione originates at the adrenals, whereas testosterone continues to be synthesized within the postmenopausal ovary. The obese individual does not necessarily have excessive estrogens but the estrogens do remain continuously unopposed.

**Pathology.** Microscopically there are two classic forms of hyperplasia, **cystic** ("Swiss cheese") and **adenomatous** ("back-to-back"). Cystic hyperplasia is a misnomer derived from the appearance of alternating dilated and narrow glands surrounded by a hyperplastic stroma; the dilated glands appeared "cystic." The only distinction from cystic atrophy is the stromal appearance that is hypocellular and fibrotic in the latter condition. Cystic hyperplasia can be focal within patches of normal secretory (progestin-dominated) endometrium. The putative explanation for this is the focal presence of progestin refractory (basalis layer) endometrium manifesting only the estrogenic effect despite an appropriate hormonal milieu. Cystic hyperplasia in itself is benign but it may progress to adenomatous hyperplasia.

cystic may → adenomatous hyperplasia

granulosa cell tumor -
rare ovarian source of excess
unopposed estrogen

*chronic irritative injury*

$\{$ Acanthosis = Focal endom. sq metaplasia

$\{$ Icthyosis = diffuse

In adenomatous hyperplasia, as the name suggests, the predominating feature is the glandular architecture. Stroma is almost nonexistent with glandular epithelium abutting directly against adjacent glands giving rise to the colloquial "back-to-back" description of this entity. If there are accompanying intracellular abnormalities it is very difficult to distinguish this entity from carcinoma-in-situ or even well-differentiated endometrial adenocarcinoma.

Thus there appears to be a progression from normal proliferative endometrium to cystic then adenomatous hyperplasia and subsequent malignancy. The documentation for such a progression is not as clear as for cervical dyplasia–CIS malignancy but is nonetheless quite strong. Persistent unopposed estrogenic predominance leads to endometrial hyperplasia that occurs before or concomitantly with adenocarcinoma.

As an aside both terms, acanthosis and uterine icthyosis, are discussed. The former refers to focal, the latter to diffuse endometrial squamous metaplasia. It arises as the result of any chronic irritative insult, e.g., irradiation, infection, or foreign body (IUD). If associated with adenoCa it is referred to as adenoacanthoma and the degree of virulence of the lesion is determined strictly by the glandular component. Should the squamous cell component undergo malignant transformation an adenosquamous cell carcinoma results (very rare). Acanthosis in itself, however, is not a harbinger of malignant disease.

***Diagnosis and Management.*** The most common presentation of endometrial hyperplasia is DUB, which should, therefore, prompt endometrial biopsy or D & C with proper pathologic examination of the scrapings. Not so much as to diagnose hyperplasia but rather to rule out possible coexistent malignancy.

When detected during childbearing years hyperplasia is often a benign manifestation of a series of anovulatory cycles that are rarely associated with a sinister underlying process. Cycling the endometrium either by providing short-term exogenous progestin (medroxyprogesterone acetate, 10 mg PO OD ×5–10d per month) or by inducing ovulation with the estrogen analogue clomiphene is sufficient therapy. If the adenomatous change appears atypical, hysterectomy is suggested because of the difficulty in distinguish-

*Atypical Aden hyperplasia → hyo*

ing atypical adenomatous hyperplasia from a well-differentiated malignancy.

## Endometrial Polyps

Polyp is a clinical term used to denote a pedunculated neoplasm, benign or malignant. Polyps are most often incidental findings on a D & C and are not consistently associated with malignancy. In the absence of secondary degenerative changes (necrosis, infection, ulceration), only a minority of endometrial polyps reach clinical attention usually through metrorrhagia. Secondary degeneration results in a foul-smelling vaginal discharge. During the childbearing years polyps can be regarded as benign lesions but postmenopausally adenomatous hyperplasia on a polyp warrants thorough D & C and any degree of atypia warrants an even more aggressive approach. Polyps and adenomatous atypia in postmenopausal women are associated with endometrial malignancy in 10% of cases. Polyps themselves very rarely undergo malignant transformation.

*D+C*

## ENDOMETRIAL CARCINOMA    *(90% Adeno CA)*

Endometrial carcinoma is the most common malignancy of the female reproductive tract. This is probably due to a true increase in incidence of endometrial cancer and the decline in incidence of cervical cancer. The endometrial epithelium is glandular, therefore, adenocarcinoma is the most common (> 90%) form of malignant disease. The average age at detection is 59 years, (i.e., postmenopausal). The actual increase in incidence is attributed to increased awareness, increased longevity, and increased use of exogenous estrogenic supplementation.

As noted in the section on hyperplasia and polyps, persistent unopposed estrogenic stimulation of the endometrium is associated with hyperplasia, which often precedes or coexists with endometrial malignancy. Conditions associated with excessive or unopposed estrogens are also overrepresented in endometrial adenocarcinoma patients. Cystic hyperplasia is benign; the adenomatous variety leads to malignancy in about 20% of cases, whereas atypical adenomatous patterns or CIS leads to malignancy in about 60% of situations.

*benign = cystic hyperplasia*

*Atypical adenomatous → malignancy*
*( or cis )                        60%*

***Pathology.*** Grossly the disease can be either diffuse or circumscribed. The former is a fungating growth that involves all or most of the endometrial surface. In the absence of myomata or pregnancy, the rate of uterine enlargement correlates with the severity of local disease. The circumscribed or focal variety of the disease involves only a small fraction of the endometrial surface.

Microscopically there is a paucity of stroma and an overabundance of glandular epithelial cells with intraluminal proliferation. Eventual obliteration of the glandular pattern occurs. An increased number of mitotic figures, large nuclei and nucleoli with prominent chromatin clumping, are suggestive of atypia. Occasionally a clear cell variant form of adenocarcinoma is noted. It may be a primary or metastatic lesion. Cytogenetic studies have failed to demonstrate aneuploidy of the malignant cells as is commonly seen in cervical malignancy.   *∅ aneuploidy*

Adenoacanthoma has already been described in the section on hyperplasia. The degree of malignancy of the lesion is determined by the glandular component. Approximately 10% of adenocarcinomas are actually adenoacanthomas. They tend to have a better prognosis than plain adenocarcinoma because the glandular component tends to be less malignant for unknown reasons. Adenosquamous cell carcinoma in which both cell types are malignant has a worse prognosis than simple adenocarcinoma. Squamous cell carcinoma of the corpus is extremely rare but carries a uniformly dismal outlook with more than 90% of patients having distant metastases at time of diagnosis.

***Histologic Grading.*** Endometrial carcinoma is one of the few instances where histologic grading does correlate with clinical outcome; perhaps more so because it parallels other prognostic factors (depth of invasion, extent of lymphatic metastases) rather than being a truly independent prognostic entity. Eighty percent of the lesions are grade 1 or 2 at diagnosis.

| Grade | Degree of Differentiation |
|---|---|
| 1 | Well differentiated |
| 2 | Moderately well differentiated |
| 3 | Poorly differentiated |

*Risk Factors: HTN, DM, Obesity, infertility*
*3/4 Post-menopausal*
*15-25% of Post-menopausal Vag bleeding att*
*to endometrial Adeno Ca.*

**Clinical.** Three quarters of the patients are postmenopausal. A previously defined subpopulation with hypertension, diabetes mellitus, obesity, and infertility were said to be at high risk of this disease. In fact documentation is only available for the latter two factors, which are often associated with persistent unopposed estrogen influence (infertility as the manifestation of repeated anovulatory cycles).

As for hyperplasia, the most common presenting complaint is abnormal periods, either postmenopausal vaginal bleeding or premenopausal hypermenorrhagia. It is estimated that between 15% and 25% of postmenopausal vaginal bleeding is attributed to endometrial adenocarcinoma. Pelvic pressure and vaginal discharge (typically serous at first, but later becoming sanguinous) may also be associated with endometrial malignancy.

**Diagnostic Investigations.** Postmenopausal vaginal bleeding implicates cervical or endometrial malignancy until proven otherwise. The initial workup is aimed at ruling out a vaginal or cervical lesion. The former by inspection; the latter by Pap smear (and biopsy if necessary).

Endometrial lesions are identified by either simple biopsy or **fractional D & C.** For the latter the cervix is biopsied, then the endocervix is biopsied, finally the uterus is sounded, the cervix dilated, and the cavity scraped. This ensures specific localization with sequential biopsies in an orderly fashion. Adenocarcinoma is usually characterized by abundant friable or necrotic endometrial scrapings ("fish-flesh appearance").

**Staging.** Staging criteria do not take into account findings at surgery so that those treated by radiotherapy alone remain comparable to surgical patients. *RT* Routine staging procedures include a fractional D & C, proctoscopy, and cystoscopy. The factors that have been found to correlate with worsening outcome are: (1) clinical stage, (2) histologic grade, (3) uterine size; (4) depth of myometrial invasion, (5) lymph node metastases, and (6) patient age. Patients with vaginal involvement at diagnosis have a worse prognosis because they tend to have less well differentiated lesions. Distant metastases seed into the peritoneum, the liver, and the lungs.

*15-25% of Postmenopausal vaginal bleeding is attributed to endometrial adenocarcinoma.*

Heyman   Packing

*Treatment.* The mainstay of therapy is surgical. Radiotherapy is a useful adjunct for selected patients. Three surgical approaches are available. Total abdominal hysterectomy with bilateral salpingo-oopherectomy (TAH with BSO) is currently the procedure of choice. Vaginal hysterectomy is suggested for those who would not withstand a longer procedure. Vaginal hysterectomy precludes exploration of the peritoneal cavity for metastases and technical difficulties with oopherectomy difficult. The most extreme approach is radical hysterectomy with pelvic lymph node dissection (seldom performed). The ovaries are resected because of a 10% incidence of gonadal involvement. TAH/BSO with resection of any grossly abnormal nodes represents a reasonable compromise.

Irradiation can be either intracavity or external. Heyman packing refers to a mode of intracavitary application of radioactive agents that achieves acceptable levels of radiation at the uterine fundus. It also provides substantial radiation to some of the pelvic nodes. Commonly a combination of 4000 rads externally and one or two subsequent internal applications of 8000 rads each (at vaginal vault) suffices. Comparison of the results of surgical and radiotherapy patients must take into account the bias in the latter patient population toward the elderly, medically ill, and more advanced disease.

Selected patients may benefit from postop internal or external radiotherapy. Inpatients with early disease radiotherapy decreases the incidence of vaginal cuff recurrences and treats pelvic lymph nodes more effectively.

Finally, progestational chemotherapy may be effective for local or distant (especially pulmonary) recurrences in up to 30% of cases.

## OVARIAN NEOPLASIA     Prognosis = f(clinical stage)

There are many classifications intended to facilitate the study and management of ovarian neoplasia. The system used in this discussion is based on the embryonic tissues that combine to give rise to the female gonad, thus a review of genitourinary tract (specifically gonadal) embryology is suggested.

There are five groups of tumors that arise primarily in the ovary from (1) the coelomic epithelium, (2) the specialized gonadal mesenchyme, (3) the germ cells, (4) the embryonic rests, (5) the nonspecialized stroma, as well as metastatic neoplasms.

*Epidemiology.* Ovarian neoplastic disorders represent ~25% of the malignancies of the female genital tract. The female gonad is obscured from physical examination, thus malignant disease tends to go unrecognized longer, unfavorably biasing the prognosis. Prognosis is most closely related to the clinical stage at diagnosis (Table 4-17). The mean 5-year survival for malignant lesions is ~20% to 30%. The mortality of ovarian malignancy exceeds that of either cervical or endometrial lesions and represents the fourth most common cause of cancer-related death in women. Risk factors identified for ovarian malignancy include nulliparity and carcinoma of the breast. Ovarian malignancy is associated with an increased risk of breast carcinoma.

*Clinical.* Signs and symptoms of ovarian carcinoma occur relatively late in the course of the disease. They include: (1) increasing abdominal girth, (2) lower abdominal heaviness or pain, (3) abnormal periods especially

**TABLE 4-17. CLINICAL STAGING FOR OVARIAN NEOPLASMS**

| Stage | Description |
|---|---|
| I | **Neoplasm limited to ovaries:**<br>(a) One ovary involved ⎫ No ascites<br>(b) Both ovaries involved ⎭<br>(c) As above but with malignant ascites |
| II | **Pelvic extension including[a]:**<br>(a) Uterus and/or fallopian tubes ⎫ No ascites<br>(b) Further pelvic extension ⎭<br>(c) As above but with malignant ascites |
| III | **Intra-abdominal or retroperitoneal extension** |
| IV | **Distant visceral metastases and/or malignant pleural effusion** |

[a]Refers to the true pelvic cavity delimited by the pelvic brim.
*Note:* Unlike endometrial adenocarcinoma, here the laparotomy findings **are** permitted to contribute to the staging process because the procedure is routinely performed whenever ovarian neoplasia is suspect.

*— exudative ascites, until proven
otherwise, means ovarian neoplasm.
— any adnexal mass*

**162**     OB/GYN NOTES

postmenopausal bleeding, and (4) pelvic thrombophlebitis. Ascities is another late finding which may complicate secondary peritoneal dissemination
or adnexal torsion. Exudative ascites in women should suggest ovarian
neoplasm until proven otherwise. Specialized gonadal stromal neoplasms of
the ovary may present with hormonal end-organ effects. As with any large
structure (ovarian neoplasm) tethered on a thin vascular pedicle (adnexa)
torsion can occur with evidence of intra-abdominal catastrophe. Rupture of
the neoplasm can also lead to clinical presentation. Hypercalcemia has been
noted even in the absence of osteolytic metastases especially with clear cell
(mesonephroid) tumors.

*$\uparrow Ca^{2+}$*

Hard, fixed, nodular masses palpated on vaginal examination are highly suggestive of neoplasia, however, the diagnosis can only be documented
by histologic examination. A mass that feels soft, elastic, and smooth is
more likely to be a benign cystic teratoma, nevertheless any adnexal mass
should be considered to be an ovarian neoplasm until proven otherwise.
Although laproscopic visualization may be helpful, biopsy obtained by this
route is often inadequate simply due to sampling error, thus the only adequate biopsy method involves formal laparotomy. The investigation of undiagnosed ascites in postmenopausal women should always include
cytologic examination of the fluid. U/S and computed tomography (CT)
imaging are useful in the initial evaluation of the lesion (the former for
diagnosing ascites and cystic tumors, the latter for detecting retroperitoneal
nodal involvement), however, their resolution is inadequate for accurate
staging.

Histologic grading assesses: (1) individual cellular maturity, (2) the
rate of cellular turnover, and (3) the arrangement of cells with respect to one
another, to give a relatively objective estimate of the degree of malignancy
for a particular lesion. For epithelial ovarian neoplasms this distinction is not
always clear leading to the formation of another group, that of ''borderline''
lesions. Prerequisite for the diagnosis of borderline lesions is the absence of
stromal invasion. Patients with borderline lesions have much longer postoperative survival than seen with frankly malignant lesions.

*Malignant* ovarian neoplasms are rare in young women. After the diagnosis of functional cyst has been excluded the most likely lesion is benign

*Borderline ⇒ absence of stromal invasion*

cystic teratoma (dermoid cyst). Ovarian neoplasms arising in childhood have an 85% chance of being benign.

## Ovarian Neoplasms of the Coelomic Epithelium

| Epithelium Type | Epithelium Resembled |
|---|---|
| Serous | Fallopian tubes |
| Endometrioid | Endometrium |
| Mucinous | Endocervix |
| Others | |
| Mesonephroid (clear cell) *90% unilateral* | |
| Brenner | |
| Mixed | |
| Unclassified epithelial tumors | |
| Undifferentiated carcinomas | |

*90% of all ovarian neopl.*

*60-70% of ovarian malig*

[ *Note:* Any of these ovarian neoplasms can occur as benign, malignant, or borderline lesions.

Ovarian neoplasms of the coelomic epithelium originate from the modified peritoneum that overlies the ovary. This tissue was formerly erroneously referred to as the "germinal" epithelium. Coelomic epithelial tumors are the single most common group of ovarian neoplasms comprising 60% to 70% of ovarian malignancies and up to 90% of all ovarian neoplasms.

Ovarian tumors arising from this tissue can resemble the epithelia of any portion of the Müllerian tract from the fallopian tubes to the vagina. (Recall that it is the coelomic epithelium that invaginates to give rise to the Müllerian duct.) Accordingly these neoplasms are subclassified by the epithelium type they resemble: (1) **serous** type (resemble fallopian tube epithelium); (2) **endometrioid** type (resemble endometrial epithelium); and (3) **mucinous** type (resemble endocervical epithelium).

**Mesonephroid (clear cell), Brenner, and mixed epithelial** tumors are also felt to originate from the coelomic epithelium. **Brenner tumors** are defined as a mixture of both epithelial and fibrous tissue components. The designation **mixed epithelial** tumor is assigned when two or more recognizable Müllerian tract epithelia are each present in sufficient quantity to prevent classification in any of the above single epithelium groups. Finally two headings are appended for those tumors that are epithelial in origin but defy further identification, listed as the **unclassified epithelial tumors and undifferentiated carcinomas.**

## Serous Type Coelomic Epithelial Neoplasms

- Cystadenoma  25% of all ovarian Tumors.
- Papillary cystadenoma  Bilateral, Psammoma Bodies
- Fibroadenoma/cystadenofibroma  - Benign. Multiloculated
- Borderline papillary cystadenocarcinoma  - >1 layer of Epith. ∅ stromal in
- Cystadenocarcinoma  ⊕ stromal invasion.  20% < 30%/o

*Benign Serous Lesions.* Grossly the **benign serous cystadenoma** is characterized by the presence of external papillomatous outgrowths. The unilocular cyst contains a thin, watery brown fluid. The inner lining of the cyst may or may not also possess papillae. If present, the lesion is referred to as a **papillary serous cystadenoma.** This subgroup frequently possesses **psammoma bodies** (also known as calcospherites) that are radiopaque calcific concretions seen within the stroma. They are thought to represent degenerated and calcified papillae. Papillary tumors have a greater incidence of bilateral involvement and also of malignant degeneration than the simple (nonpapillary) cystadenomas.

Microscopically one sees a simple cuboidal or columnar epithelium (which may or may not be ciliated) encasing the serous fluid. If this lining is composed of a single layer the lesion is clearly benign. Serous cystadenomas represent 25% of all ovarian tumors. This entity tends to present in early adulthood, in the third or fourth decade. It is a bilateral lesion in 50% of cases and undergoes malignant degeneration in up to 40% of cases.

**Fibroadenoma,** a variant form of serous tumor, is formed by invaginations of coelomic epithelium surrounded by hyperplastic connective tissue. **Cystadenofibroma** are similar structures in which the coelomic epithelium undergoes cystic degeneration. The cysts are multilocular and always possess papillae, however, the lining tissue is the same serous epithelium described previously. Both of these entities are usually benign.

*Papillary serous cystadenoma = psammoma bodies*
*↳ Bilateral involvement common*

*Serous Borderline Papillary Cystadenocarcinoma.* This name is applied to papillary cystadenomas in which, at least focally, more than a single layer of epithelium is observed to line the papillae. Although this does not make the lesion perforce frankly malignant it is a histopathologic trait more often associated with malignant than with benign behavior. Qualitative cellular traits suggestive of malignancy (e.g., atypia) are also observed. There must be no stromal invasion by the epithelium. Loose cell clusters floating in the cyst and psammoma bodies are common.

→     Up to 50% of borderline lesions are stage 1 at diagnosis, whereas frankly malignant lesions are more often disseminated (> 75%). Patients are often asymptomatic and 20% are under the age of 30 years. Despite the fact that a large number of individuals with this form of neoplasm have metastatic lesions, surgical resection of the primary is associated with a prolonged survival.          *20% < 30 yrs age*

*Serous Cystadenocarcinoma.* Such lesions are histologically overtly malignant with epithelial invasion of the stroma. They are more common than their mucinous counterpart and almost always papillated. Ovarian tumors are notoriously variegated in microscopic appearance, thus multiple sections must be taken if malignancy is to be excluded with any degree of confidence.          *Serous > mucinous CA*
                                              *CA*

## Mucinous Type

- Cystadenoma  *very large. Broad ligament*
- Cystadenocarcinoma

*Benign Mucinous Cystadenoma.*   These lesions may be very large (e.g., 35 kg). Grossly they are irregularly lobulated, smooth-surfaced, bluewhite tumors. The wall of the tumor is thin and translucent. Adhesions that form are inflammatory and not local metastases. Mucinous cystadenomas are usually suspended by narrow highly vascular pedicles to the broad ligament.

Although this lesion is as common as serous cystadenoma, it differs in

*(incidence) M. cystadenoma ≅ S. cystadenoma*

*(size)  mucinous > serous*

*mucinous cystadeno CA rarely bilateral*
*Borderline lesions - only occassionally bilateral (10%)*

several respects. Mucinous cystadenomas are: (1) rarely bilateral, (2) often multiloculated cysts, (3) larger in size, and (4) exhibit bimodal age distribution being most common in the third and fifth decades. The presence of papillae increases the likelihood of malignant degeneration. The fluid contained in the cysts is clear and viscid. Microscopically a simple columnar epithelium (picket-fence appearance) lines the cystic cavities. Goblet cells may or may not also be present.

There is a significant incidence of concurrent dermoid cyst and mucinous cystadenoma (5%). This has lead to the theory that one or the other lesion arises from its mate by a metaplastic process.

*Borderline Mucinous Cystadenocarcinoma.* These tumors are not distinguishable grossly from frank malignancies. The stromal integrity is not breached by the epithelium. In addition, although there is stratification of the epithelium, it should not exceed three layers to qualify as a borderline lesion. There may be a great amount of variability in the degree of anaplasia seen with a tumor but the prognosis is best predicted by the least mature region. Borderline mucinous cystadenocarcinoma is only occasionally bilateral (10%), thus unilateral salpingo-oophorectomy (USO) with contralateral ovarian biopsy is sufficient initial intervention.

*Pseudomyxoma Peritoneii.* Pseudomyxoma peritoneii can complicate rupture of a benign mucinous cystadenoma. Diffuse peritoneal dissemination produces copious amounts of viscid mucous requiring repeat laparotomy for drainage. It is regarded as a form of low-grade malignant degeneration. An indolent but nonetheless progressive clinical deterioration is observed. Drainage of undiagnosed ovarian cysts should, therefore, not be attempted within the peritoneum.

*Malignant Cystadenocarcinoma.* Malignant cystadenocarcinoma results when its benign counterpart undergoes malignant degeneration, which occurs in 5% to 10% of cases. The malignancy may involve the cyst in its entirety or only focally.

Both stromal infiltration and stratification of the lining epithelium in excess of three layers are observed microscopically. The epithelium retains

*— Endometrioid lesions of the ovaries*
*assoc c̄ endometrial malignancy in*
*✗ (20%) of cases.*
*— Mesonephroid CA of ovary assoc c̄*
*Pelvic endometriosis.* **GENERAL GYNECOLOGY 167**

its ability to secrete mucous with multiple collections of gelatinous material found throughout the tumor.

***Endometrioid Type.*** Microscopically these neoplasms resemble adenocarcinoma or adenoacanthoma of the uterine corpus. Subtypes include:

- Cystadenoma
- Cystadenocarcinoma *20% c̄ endometrial malig. 1/3 bilateral involvement*
- Acanthoadenocarcinoma *c̄ squamous metaplasia*

**Endometrioid cystadenoma** is a rare, benign lesion. The more common **malignant endometrioid cystadenocarcinoma** may also display regions of squamous metaplasia in which case it is referred to as an **acanthoadenocarcinoma.** Endometrioid lesions are frequently cystic and ✓ possess papillae. They can be associated with concurrent clear cell (mesonephroid), serous, mucinous, and endometrial malignancies (the latter as often as 20%). Endometrioid cystadenocarcinoma frequently (33%) involves ✗ the ovaries bilaterally.

Prognosis for this lesion is generally poor. The rare mixed mesodermal tumor of the ovary is probably a variant form of the endometrioid malignancy containing both epithelial and stromal components.

***Mesonephroid Type (Clear Cell Tumor).*** Also known as clear cell tumors, these lesions can be cystic or solid and classically have a glomeruluslike ✗ appearance under the microscope. Mesonephroid ovarian carcinoma is usually (> 90%) a unilateral lesion. It can be cystic, solid, or a combination of both. Mesonephroid tumors are freely mobile but are often ruptured during attempted excision. They occur most often in the fifth and sixth decades. Nulliparity may represent a risk factor for developing this lesion.
*associated c̄ Pelvic endometriosis*

***Brenner Tumor.*** Brenner tumors are fibroepithelial lesions that differ from the serous cystadenofibroma in that the epithelial component is squamous rather than cuboidal. Brenner tumors are most often a benign, unilateral, ✗ postmenopausal disease. In this respect it is quite similar to ovarian thecoma. Furthermore, both thecoma and Brenner tumors, as well as ovarian fibromas, can be associated with ascites and unilateral pleural effu-

*✗ Brenner Tumor = squamous epithelium*

*Meigs Syndrome*
① Brenners
② ovarian Fibroma
③ ovarian Thecoma

sions (**Meigs' syndrome**). Brenner tumors and mucinous cystadenomas frequently coexist.

## Ovarian Neoplasms of the Specialized Gonadal Mesenchyme

By definition ovarian neoplasms of the specialized gonadal mesenchyme are lesions that are composed of female gonadal mesenchyme. Note that although they arise from the stroma (or mesenchyme), they can possess components that resemble descendants of the coelomic epithelium (sertoli and granulosa cells). Tumors of the ovary that develop from the specialized gonadal mesenchyme can be either benign or malignant. The benign entities are in fact not truly neoplastic; they are cystic.

The truly neoplastic entities are often functional, that is, they often produce sex hormones appropriate for the cell type of the tumor. This trait permits further subclassification of the neoplasms into those that produce female, male, or a mixture of both varieties of sex hormones. The female sex hormone cell tumors produce hormones in up to 85% of cases, (Table 4-18).

### Benign Cystic Lesions     *Bilateral*

- Follicle cysts (single or multiple)  *Bilateral*
- Corpus luteum cyst  *unilateral*
- Theca–lutein cyst  *Bilateral, during Preg, excessive hCG.*

*Single Follicle Cysts.* Single follicle cysts develop from atreitic follicles that become overdistended with serous fluid after they have failed to ovulate. Microscopically one sees a central cyst surrounded by granulosa and theca cells.

They are more frequent in the peripubescent age group. If the lesion is

TABLE 4-18. FUNCTIONAL NEOPLASTIC LESIONS

| Female | Male | Mixed |
|---|---|---|
| Thecoma | Leydig (hilus) cell | Gynandroblastoma |
| Granulosa cell[a] | Sertoli-Leydig[a] | |

[a]Although these tumors arise from specialized gonadal stroma they may possess components that resemble coelomic epithelium derivatives.

detected as an incidental finding on pelvic examination (adnexal mass) simple reexamination within 8 to 10 weeks is sufficient in the peripubertal age group. In older women a shorter delay interval is suggested (6 weeks). In the postmenopausal age group the incidence of more sinister lesions warrants immediate surgical intervention. Surgery should be extirpative, no attempt should be made to aspirate the cyst in situ because of the potential risk of dissemination of malignant cells.

*Multiple Follicle Cysts.* Pathologically multiple follicle cysts are characterized as bilaterally enlarged polycystic ovaries with a thickened tunica albuginea (typical of anovulatory ovaries). Furthermore, the theca interna is notably hyperplastic. This form of ovary is associated with the polycystic ovary disease (PCOD) or Stein-Leventhal syndrome. Therapy consists of clomiphene citrate or wedge resection of the ovary.

*Corpus Luteum Cysts.* The corpus luteum is usually a cystic structure, however, if it experiences continued growth or hemorrhage within the cyst it becomes pathologically enlarged and detectable on pelvic examination as an adnexal mass. The cyst is seen to contain blood, serous coagulum, and connective tissue linked by luteinized (fat laden) granulosa and theca interna cells. The lipid within these cells is used in the synthesis of progesterone and ultimately sex steroids. The production of sex steroids leads to pituitary suppression and amenorrhea-simulating pregnancy.

Clinically this entity presents with secondary amenorrhea followed by a scant persistent vaginal blood loss. The patient may also complain of unilateral pelvic pain and a small tender adnexal mass. The only therapeutic modality available is conservative surgical excision, however, surgery is delayed as long as the clinical situation permits, (i.e., pain and hemorrhage remain tolerable).

*Theca–Lutein Cysts.* Theca–Lutein cysts are a rare variant form of corpus luteum cysts that occur during pregnancy and are almost always bilateral. They are frequently associated with excessive HCG levels, e.g., molar pregnancy.

Microscopically the cyst is lined by luteinized theca interna cells of mesenchymal origin (and rarely also by luteinized granulosa cells). Thecal

*T-L cysts – Bilateral. Assoc c̄ moles*

Granulosa Cell Tumors — Call-Exner Bodies (immature Primordial Follicles)
⊛ estrogen producing
— 15-25% of Postmen g cell Tumors assoc c concurrent endometrial CA

✱ cells are <u>LH</u> responsive, thus after the associated trophoblastic tissue (source of <u>HCG</u> that possesses primarily LH activity) is removed the cysts usually resolve.

Theca–lutein cysts are most often an incidental asymptomatic finding that requires (no) specific attention. Should hemorrhage into the cyst or into the peritoneum occur, surgical removal is indicated.

## Neoplastic Lesions

*Granulosa Cell Tumor.* Granulosa cell tumors are neoplasms that arise from the <u>early ovarian stroma</u> and vary in size from several grams to several kilograms. Grossly they appear to be friable gray–yellow solid structures with occasional cystic cavities. Microscopically the constituent cells resemble granulosa cells. <u>Luteinization</u> may occur on occasion. **Call-Exner** bodies or immature primordial follicles are associated with this variety of ovarian lesion.

The etiology is unknown, however, such neoplasms may be associated with Peutz-Jegher's syndrome (intestinal hamartomas, mucosal and cutaneous melanin spots; autosomal dominant) or with <u>pregnancy luteomas</u>. The latter refers to focal stromal luteinization not uncommonly seen during pregnancy. The luteoma is separate from the corpus luteum proper. Although this entity usually regresses spontaneously after pregnancy ends it may represent the primordium of the granulosa cell tumor.

Granulosa cell neoplasms account for (10%) of ovarian malignancy and can occur at any age. They often produce (estrogen,) thus, in addition to increased abdominal girth and pelvic pain, they may produce hormonally induced signs and symptoms. The clinically significant markers of excess estrogen levels vary with respect to patient age:

| Prepubertal | Reproductive Age | Postmenopausal |
|---|---|---|
| Isosexual precocious puberty, premature menarche, breast enlargement, pubic hair | Hypermenorrhea | Recurrent menses Proliferative endo-metrium on biopsy |

Granulosa cell tumors are low grade malignancies with a (50%) 20-year survival. High estrogen levels associated with granulosa cell tumors increase

Tend to recur more than 5 yrs @ initial Dx. Malig Potential impossible to predict histologically. Recurrences have been reported as late as 33 yrs @ original Dx.

the risk of endometrial adenocarcinoma. Fifteen percent to 25% of feminizing postmenopausal granulosa cell tumors are associated with concurrent endometrial malignancy.

Therapeutic intervention is limited to surgical resection. The patients are often young and the lesions small and unilateral, thus USO usually suffices.

*Thecoma.* Thecomas usually possess no coelomic epithelial components and they are usually unilateral, postmenopausal, and almost always benign. In this respect **thecomas** are very similar to **fibromas** of the ovary, which arise from the nonspecific ovarian stroma. They also can both be associated with **Meigs' syndrome** (nonmalignant hydrothorax and ascites). Thecoma, however, is capable of producing estrogen and, therefore, can cause signs and symptoms of excess estrogen (see above).

Although unilateral the estrogen production often results in diffuse contralateral thecomatosis (nonneoplastic predominance of thecal cells). On microscopy these lesions are seen to contain spindle-shaped cells separated by connective tissue bands that may or may not be hyalinized. The cells are densely lipid-laden as suggested by the presence of intracellular doubly refractile fat on microscopy.

Surgical resection and histologic examination documents the type of tumor and has occasionally been associated with resolution of Meigs' syndrome.

*Leydig (Hilus) Cell Tumor.* Leydig cell tumor is an extremely rare form of ovarian neoplasia. It is most often a benign, virilizing, postmenopausal neoplasm. Hirsuitism can occur in addition to menstrual dysfunction and infertility (the latter only if premenopausal). Virilization results from testosterone secretion by the tumor.

Histologically, visualization of rodlike **Reinke's albuminoid crystals** are pathognomonic, however, they are not essential for the diagnosis. Surgical excision provides relief from the virilization.

*Sertoli-Leydig (Arrhenoblastoma) Cell Tumor.* Sertoli-Leydig cell tumors of the ovary are also rare, virilizing ovarian neoplasms. The color, size, and consistency of these neoplasms are variable. They tend to be solid with minimal cystic degeneration. Microscopically Sertoli-Leydig cell tumors are variable from highly differentiated forms strongly resembling normal seminiferous tubule architecture to poorly differentiated forms in which there is no detectable histologic organization. Arrhenoblastomas are low-grade malignancies.

Sertoli-Leydig neoplasms arise in the third decade and tend to manifest in two clinical phases. The initial phase consists of **defeminization,** or subtraction of female secondary sex characteristics (amennorhea, breast atrophy, decreased subcutaneous fat); the latter is marked by **virilization,** the addition of male secondary sex traits (clitoral hypertrophy, hirsuitism, deepening voice).

Unilateral salpingo-oophorectomy is usually sufficient therapy. This tumor is rarely bilateral. Chemotherapy may be required for extraovarian metastases. The defeminizing features resolve quickly, however, the virilizing traits may not revert.

*Gynandroblastoma.* Gynandroblastoma is an extremely rare ovarian neoplasm that contains elements resembling granulosa, Sertoli, and Leydig cells mixed or adjacent to one another. The clinical manifestations are similarly an unpredictable mixture of virilization and excess feminization (e.g., endometrial hyperplasia). They are treated like Sertoli-Leydig cell tumors.

## Ovarian Neoplasms of the Primordial Germ Cells

This section deals with neoplastic ovarian lesions that arise from descendants of the primordial germ cells. The germ cells originate from yolk sac endoderm at about the fourth week of gestation and subsequently migrate to the developing gonad. Arrest of these primordia anywhere along this migration (with subsequent malignant degeneration) accounts for the ectopy that can be observed with ovarian germ cell tumors (Fig. 4-5).

*Dysgerminoma.* Dysgerminoma is the most common malignant germ cell tumor of the ovary. It lacks any teratomatous elements, and carries with it the best prognosis of all malignant ovarian neoplasms with the exception of the borderline epithelial lesions. Dysgerminoma is the female equivalent to the male testicular seminoma. It occurs most commonly in the second and

Dysgerminoma (♀) = seminoma (♂)

Most radiosensitive

3-5%

75% are stage 1 at Dx

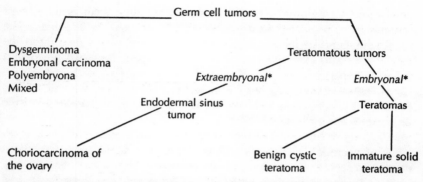

*, Embryonal tumors are composed of tissues that resemble portions of the embryo, whereas extraembryonal tumors are composed of extraembryonic germ cell derivatives.

**Figure 4-5.** Ovarian neoplasms of the primordial germ cells.

third decades and may be associated with other coexistent germ cell malignancies. Dysgerminoma represents ~3% to 5% of all ovarian malignancies. The germ cells from which this lesion develops are neither feminizing nor virilizing. Dysgerminomas are more common in maldeveloped gonads e.g., Turner's syndrome and male pseudohermaphrodites with streak gonads.

Dysgerminomas are usually solid unilateral gray-pink lesions of rubbery consistency. Although the smaller tumors appear to have a thick capsule, it is easily breached with subsequent spread. The microscopic picture is one of nests of large, ovoid polygonal cells separated by hyalinized connective tissue septae.

The degree of malignancy is variable but if the capsule of the lesion is transgressed the prognosis is significantly worsened. Other factors suggesting poor prognosis include: (1) bilaterality, (2) occurrence during some form of pregnancy, (3) concurrent teratomatous neoplasm, and (4) spillage of tumor contents intraperitoneally during the surgical procedure.

The treatment advocated for stage 1 (localized to the ovaries) lesions is USO. Seventy-five percent of dysgerminomas are stage 1 at diagnosis. For any higher stage TAH/BSO with adjunctive radiotherapy is indicated (**dysgerminoma is the most radiosensitive solid ovarian neoplasm**).

*αFP and βHCG*
*Never Bilateral*
*⊕ syncytiotrophoblast*
*∅ cytotrophoblast*

*Embryonal Carcinoma.* Relatively uncommon, this tumor is the female counterpart of testicular embryonal carcinoma in men. In addition to the usual complaints of increasing abdominal girth and pelvic discomfort the patient may also experience signs and symptoms of isosexual precocious puberty, hypermenorrhea, and other manifestations of excess estrogen. **Plasma alpha-fetoprotein and beta-HCG** may be elevated with this tumor. Embryonal carcinoma is a misnomer because this lesion is not one of the embryonal germ cell tumor group.

Grossly the external surface is usually smooth with multiple soft regions of necrotic degeneration. There are foci of highly undifferentiated cells interspersed with foci of identifiable syncytiotrophoblast. Cytotrophoblast is absent which distinguishes embryonal carcinoma from true choriocarcinoma. Embryonal carcinoma has never been reported to be bilateral, thus USO with triple-agent adjuvant chemotherapy is indicated.

### Extraembryonal Teratomatous Germ Cell Tumors

*Pain*

*Endodermal Sinus Tumor.* Of the malignant germ cell tumors, the endodermal sinus tumor is second in frequency only to dysgerminoma. This highly malignant entity almost always presents before the age of 45 years. It is most often unilateral with up to 75% being discretely palpable. Unlike other ovarian neoplasms the most common presenting complaint is pain. Note that up to one third of endodermal sinus tumors rupture preoperatively or intraoperatively. *Schiller-Duval Bodies*

Pathologic examination reveals a large necrotic mass composed of cuboidal cells with a loose stroma. The sinuses surround structures referred to as pseudopapillae, the entire tumor staining strongly for **alpha-fetoprotein.** Alpha-fetoprotein is a protein of endodermal yolk sac origin. Serum alpha-fetoprotein levels are also elevated.

The high degree of malignancy of this tumor is reflected by a 93% 2-year mortality. Management usually involves a combination of surgery and postoperative chemotherapy.

*Choriocarcinoma of the Ovary.* Choriocarcinoma in the ovary is most often related to gestational trophoblastic disease, but it can arise indepen-

Dermoid
① most common germ cell Tumor
② most common that presents before
   age 20
GENERAL GYNECOLOGY    175
⑤ Thyroid Tissue (10%) = struma ovarii
④ Carcinoids can arise de Novo.

dently (very rare). Primary ovarian choriocarcinoma is highly malignant. Furthermore it is relatively unresponsive to chemotherapy.

*Benign Cystic Teratoma.* Benign cystic teratoma is also known as **dermoid cyst** because of the early observation that skin and skin appendages were frequently present in the tumor. Benign cystic teratoma is the most common germ cell tumor. It accounts for 10% of all ovarian neoplasms. *20-25* Benign cystic teratoma is the most common ovarian neoplasm that presents before the age of 20 years, the peak incidence being between 20 and 40 years of age.

Dermoids are usually composed of a thick-walled capsule of squamous epithelium with skin appendages surrounding a unilocular cyst full of de-squamated cells as well as the cheesy products of capsular wall glands. Grossly the contents appear greasy yellow with a fluid consistency at body temperature becoming pultaceous shortly after surgical removal.

In keeping with the fact that this is an embryonal tumor, all three primordial tissues (endoderm, mesoderm, ectoderm) may be represented. Frequently a single embryonal tissue dominates the tumor contents: (1) choroid plexus and CSF; (2) teeth (50%) and other bony remnants; (3) cartilage; (4) neural tissue; (5) gastrointestinal mucosa; or (6) thyroid tissue *10%* (the rare **struma ovarii** variant that can cause thyrotoxicosis). Regardless of the predominantly cystic nature of dermoids there is usually an area of solid tissue within the capsule that contains the remaining embryonal tissues.

*2/3 are benign*

Carcinoid tumors are usually GI tract primaries that can metastasize to the ovary but they can also arise de novo in a dermoid. Such carcinoids are equally capable of giving rise to carcinoid syndrome (episodic flushing, wheezing and diarrhea).

Complications of benign cystic teratomas include torsion with or without rupture of the cyst and rarely hemolytic anemia (which may resolve on extirpation of the primary lesion). Dermoid rupture is uncommon because of the thick capsule. Torsion is the most common complication of benign ovarian cysts.

Malignant degeneration is rare, occurring in < 3% of cases. The majority of malignancies evolve from the ectodermal component and are therefore carcinomas either squamous cell (80%) or adenocarcinoma (7%). Prognosis

⑤ Complications
   - hemolytic disease (rare)
   - Torsion (common)

is related to the integrity of the capsule and the existence of extragonadal involvement. If the capsule is intact and there are no distant metastases the 5-year survival may be as high as 80%.

Surgical resection usually suffices as therapy. Benign cystic teratomas are often pedunculated being suspended anteriorly from the broad ligament. This facilitates resection of the lesion and preservation of the ovary. Although contralateral involvement (15%) is usually grossly apparent biopsy is still advisable even if the contralateral ovary appears grossly normal.

*Solid Teratoma.* Solid teratoma is also known as immature or malignant teratoma, contains one or all of the three primordial embryonic tissues. Solid teratomas are somewhat more common in children and young adults. **Beta-HCG, alpha-fetoprotein, and carcinoembryonic antigen** are plasma markers associated with this lesion. The degree of malignancy best correlates with the histologic grade of the primary lesion. Solid teratoma is usually unilateral and therefore USO represents sufficient surgical intervention. Postoperative adjuvant chemotherapy is helpful. Radiotherapy is of little benefit.

## Ovarian Neoplasms of the Embryonic Rests

*Adrenal Rest Tumor (Lipid Cell Tumor, Adrenal Tumor of the Ovary).* Adrenal rest tumor is a rare entity that belongs functionally with "male" germ cell tumors of the ovary because of its tendency to virilize. On histologic examination the adrenal rest tumor has cells that resemble those of the adrenal cortex, luteinized granulosa/theca interna, or Leydig's (hilus) cells. This histologic appearance is not sufficiently similar to any of the above tissues to be classified a such.

Grossly they are large, unilateral, solid tumors that can occur at any age. They tend to virilize or at least defeminize.

## Ovarian Neoplasms of the Nonspecialized Stroma

Ovarian neoplasms of the nonspecialized stroma include fibromas, angiomas, leiomyomas, and rarely sarcomas. The majority of these lesions are unilateral, benign, solid, postmenopausal lesions, usually detected as incidental findings on pelvic examination. Ovarian fibroma can be associated

*Fibromas = Meigs Syndrome*

with **Meigs' syndrome.** Grossly fibromas appear as small white–yellow solid nodules on the surface of the ovary. Microscopically there may be evidence of mesenchymal components other than simple fibrocytes, e.g., muscle, cartilage.

## METASTATIC TUMORS TO THE OVARY *from breast or GI tract*

Metastatic lesions account for only 6% of all ovarian neoplasia and may originate from virtually any organ. Most commonly spread occurs from the breast or GI tract. The only GU tract malignancy that spreads to the ovaries with any degree of frequency is endometrial adenocarcinoma.

The **Krukenberg** tumor warrants specific attention. Histologically the characteristic finding is the presence of "**signet ring**" cells named for the eccentric displacement of the nuclei. Signet ring cells are usually surrounded by reactive proliferation of ovarian stroma. Krukenberg tumors of the ovary may occur with primary lesions at: (1) the stomach or intestine, (2) the breast, or (3) the endometrium. Krukenberg's tumors are bilateral in over 50% of cases and may possess the potential to synthesize sex steroids with clinically evident effect.

*Treatment.* Because clinical presentation is late, as many as 65% of ovarian neoplasms are widely disseminated (stage 3 or worse) at initial diagnosis. Peritoneal dissemination results from direct contact and lymphatic spread. Extragonadal spread defies complete surgical extirpation, nonetheless, low-grade or borderline lesions benefit from surgical "debulking". Reports vary somewhat but the general consensus is that tumor residua less than 2 cm in diameter are correlated with significantly prolonged survivals.

Total abdominal hysterectomy and bilateral salpingo-oophorectomy is the procedure of choice for most malignant ovarian lesions. If, however, the disease is stage 1(a) and the patient wishes to retain reproductive capacity, USO with contralateral biopsy can be performed. Patients require close follow-up and possibly even prophylatic removal of the remaining ovary once reproductive goals are attained.

With the exception of specialized gonadal stromal tumors ovarian malignancies carry a poor prognosis. Postoperative adjuvant combination chemotherapy is often required. Radiotherapy is less helpful because most ovarian malignancies are widely disseminated at the time of diagnosis and most local lesions are relatively radioresistant. A "second look" laparotomy performed several weeks after initial surgery and adjuvant chemotherapy is intended to establish the combined efficacy of therapy and remove any further residua amenable to resection. Laparoscopy is inadequate for this purpose because fibrotic adhesions obscure full visualization.

As many as 33% of ovarian neoplasms are detected during pregnancy. If ovarian neoplasia is diagnosed during pregnancy, surgery is delayed until after the first trimester unless an acute abdominal catastrophe occurs, e.g., torsion. The timing of surgery is dependent on tumor size, position, and growth rate, as well as on the stage of gestation. If there is substantial evidence to indicate that the lesion is frankly malignant, surgery should not be delayed. Otherwise, a midtrimester unilateral salpingo-oophorectomy (USO) is suggested.

✳ ⅓ of ovarian neoplasms are detected during pregnancy

# 5

# Reproductive Gynecology

## PUBERTY

Puberty is that period during which fertility is attained; secondary sex characteristics (breast development, pubic and axillary hair growth, enlargement of external genitalia, and body fat redistribution) develop and axial skeletal growth is completed. In women this usually occurs during late childhood or early adolescence.

In 75% of cases the first physical evidence on incipient puberty is thelarche (breast development, estrogen-mediated), followed by adrenarche (adrenal androgen-mediated appearance of pubic and axillary hair), axial skeletal growth spurt, and menarche (normal duration of this process is ~2½ years). In another 25% of individuals adrenarche precedes thelarche. Tanner has described stages of breast and pubic hair development during puberty thus facilitating objective reproducible observations. Suffice it to say, however, that: (1) menarche usually attends Tanner stage IV of breast development and (2) secondary sex traits normally develop in synchrony.

The first detectable hormonal change in puberty is the episodic secretion of luteinizing hormone (LH) during REM sleep. This may be due to declining central sensitivity to gonadal steroid feedback inhibition. As gonadotropin levels rise, the ovaries produce more estrogen. Eventually estrogen levels are sufficient to induce positive feedback stimulation of LH secretion giving rise to the midcycle ovulatory LH surge. Thereafter, luteal phases occur with the menstrual cycles and thus, detectable elevations of progesterone. Adrenal androgen production increases throughout puberty.

**179**

Prolactin and testosterone levels also rise gradually throughout puberty (the latter is of minimal significance in women).

Puberty is often accompanied by psychic maturation with an increase in abstract ideation and a search for identity. Fertility at this point represents, at best a hindrance, and at worst a threat of unwanted pregnancy. Although nothing can surpass reasoned parental counseling at this stage of life, physicians may be called upon to augment or fulfill this task. Such counseling should include a candid discussion of the advisability of contraception if the patient intends to be sexually active.

Delayed pubertal development is defined and described in the section discussing primary amenorrhea. Precocious puberty is defined as the development of secondary sex traits **or** menses before 8 years of age (girls). Heterosexual precocious puberty is an indication of significant organic dysfunction. Isosexual precocity is divided into two categories, **complete** (ovulatory cycles and synchronous development of secondary sex traits) and **incomplete** (isolated development of particular secondary sex traits or menarche without ovulatory cycles). Precocity of any form is always associated with initial acceleration of axial growth but diminution of the ultimate height achieved such that it rarely exceeds 150 cm.

Although many conditions can be associated with complete isosexual precocious puberty (discussed later), its chief significance is that the patient is fertile, necessitating counseling and possibly other contraceptive precautions. Incomplete isosexual precocity can be more ominous, being on occasion associated with ovarian or adrenal malignancies. Benign conditions that should be considered include: (1) premature thelarche, i.e., unilateral or bilateral transient (several months), breast enlargement usually occurring before 2 years of age; (2) premature pubarche in the absence of virilization or other secondary sex traits (note that in 25% of cases normal puberty commences with adrenarche; (3) exposure to exogenous hormone containing agents including oral contraceptive pills, vitamin formulations, and cosmetics (see Medical Letter 1985;277:54–5); (4) foreign body (when the sole problem is premature menarche).

Investigations include: visual field examination and fundoscopy (papilledema) for the possible detection of expanding pituitary lesions; abdominal examination for adrenal or gonadal masses; gonadotropin, testosterone, adrenal androgen (heterosexual precocity), estrogen, beta-HCG (ectopic chorionic hamartomas), and thyroid hormone levels. Complete isosexual precocity is characterized by an elevation in serum gonadotropins, whereas incomplete precocity is usually associated with abnormally low gonadotropin levels.

The goals of treatment of isosexual precocious puberty are twofold: (1) to stave off further sexual development, fertility, and the possible psychologic harm that may be incurred and (2) to preserve the growth potential of the axial skeleton. The former can be achieved with medroxyprogesterone acetate (100 to 200 mg IM q1–2wk) or cyproterone acetate (either 50 to 200 mg/m²/d PO or 100 to 250 mg/m² IM q2–4wk). Medroxyprogesterone may be complicated by glucose intolerance, weight gain, and mild to moderate hypertension due to its glucocorticoid and mineralocorticoid properties. There are presently no effective means of preserving skeletal growth potential.

## MENOPAUSE   *cessation of menses. → 1° ovarian insufficiency*

Menopause, defined as the cessation of menses, occurs at an average age of 50 years in North America. The climacteric refers to the endocrine, somatic, and psychic changes associated with the loss of fertility and may occur over the subsequent 1 to 2 years. Menopause is a manifestation of primary ovarian insufficiency. The decline in estrogen feedback inhibition on the pituitary results in increased gonadotropin secretion. Increased follicle-stimulating hormone (FSH) levels results in shortening of the follicular stage of the menstrual cycle with a further decline in the estrogen level until it fails to induce the midcycle ovulatory LH surge. After several anovulatory cycles, ovarian parenchymal steroid synthesis ceases as does uterine bleeding. The ovarian stroma continues to produce androstenedione that is converted to estrone within peripheral adipose tissue, thus the postmenopausal individual is not totally devoid of female sex hormones.   *↑FSH*   *↓est*

Approximately one quarter of the menopausal female population has symptoms severe enough to warrant medical attention. Symptoms that arise from menopause occur either early or late (Table 5-1). The anxieties attendant upon the loss of reproductive capacity and their physical and psychologic repercussions constitute a secondary group of symptoms.

*androstenedione → estrone*

**TABLE 5-1. MENOPAUSAL SYMPTOMS**

| Early | Late |
|---|---|
| Hot flushing (vasomotor instability) | Dyspareunia/urethritis (genitourinary atrophy) |
| Irregular menses | Short stature/kyphosis/bone pain (osteoporosis) |
| Insomnia | ? Atherosclerotic heart disease |

*[handwritten: FSH levels > 100 IU/L]*

Laboratory confirmation of the diagnosis of menopause (primary ovarian insufficiency) rests on the documentation of elevated FSH levels (> 100 IU/L) in the blood. LH blood levels cannot be relied on because the same levels (> 75 IU/L) can be associated with the midcycle ovulatory surge. FSH levels should be repeated to ensure the diagnosis. In the case of premature menopause, an ovarian biopsy may also be indicated for the same purpose (see amenorrhea section).   *[handwritten: α-agonist]*

Treatment with estrogen or clonidine (a central alpha-agonist agent with potent anticholinergic effects) may be indicated for moderate to severe early menopausal symptoms. Estrogen when used in this context represents replacement therapy for the failing ovary.

Contraindications to estrogen therapy include:

- Pregnancy
- Undiagnosed uterine bleeding
- Estrogen-dependent neoplasia
- Active liver disease
- Thromboembolic disease

Note that the following dosage regimen may require alteration due to the wide patient-to-patient variation in response to estrogens:

Conjugated estrogens   1.25 mg PO OD × 2 wk
then 0.625 mg PO OD × 3 wk ⎫
no meds × 1 wk ⎬ × 3 mo
then 0.3 mg PO OD × 3–6 mo ⎭

If symptoms reappear while the estrogen is being tapered the dosage should be increased; minor side effects (including nausea, emesis, breast distension) merit dosage reduction and major adverse reactions (undiagnosed uterine bleeding, estrogen dependent neoplasia) warrant discontinuation of estrogen therapy. Whenever long-term estrogen therapy is being contemplated it must be cycled with occasional progestational influence to decrease the likelihood of inducing endometrial adenocarcinoma. Patients may refuse this form of therapy because they no longer wish to endure continued menses.

Clonidine (0.05 mg PO BID for 2 to 4 weeks) acts to increase vasomotor stability by its sympatholytic properties. Although less effective in relieving flushing episodes it does not increase the risk of endometrial neoplasia. Clonidine may cause atropinism (dry mouth and eyes, urinary retention, constipation) and hypotension. Overdosage produces atropinic delerium with fever and tachycardia. Abrupt discontinuation has sometimes been associated with rebound hypertension requiring resumption of the agent.

Dyspareunia and urethritis due to genitourinary atrophy respond well to vaginal suppository formulations of estrogens. The development, or acceleration, of atherosclerosis during postmenopausal life is still an issue of controversy.

Postmenopausal osteoporosis is related etiologically to increased bone resorption due to estrogen deficiency, dietary intake that is poor in calcium and rich in phosphates, and suboptimal peak bone density. Processes that interfere with adequate sun exposure or vitamin D intake will also exacerbate bone demineralization.

The use of estrogen for the prevention of excessive bone resorption is instituted and carried out according to the therapeutic principles outlined previously. Although some advocate prophylactic use of estrogen it is difficult to define the subpopulation of patients at risk of postmenopausal osteoporosis who would benefit most from such intervention. Other preventive and therapeutic measures include: adequate exercise and sun exposure, $CaCO_3$ 2.5 g/d PO, and a low phosphate-, calcium-rich diet. In addition to estrogen, vitamin D 50,000 units PO q2wk $\times$ 4mo, can be given to those individuals with more pronounced symptoms.

# AMENORRHEA   *must R/o pregnancy 1st*

Amenorrhea is the absence or abnormal stoppage of the menses. Primary amenorrhea is defined as: (1) the absence of a menstrual period, growth spurt, and secondary sexual traits by 14 years of age; (2) the absence of a menstrual period by 16 years of age regardless of the other features of puberty. Secondary amenorrhea is the absence of menses for an interval equal to three normal periods (for that particular patient) or 6 months in a woman who was previously menstruating.

The initial diagnosis which must be considered is pregnancy. More likely to present as secondary amenorrhea, pregnancy may be the cause of primary amenorrhea also.

The occurrence of menstruation is documented by the presence of visible bleeding. For this to occur all facets or compartments of the female genitourinary tract must be intact. Compartment-I refers to an intact outflow tract from the steroid responsive endometrial surface to the vaginal orifice; compartment-II refers to gonadotropin responsive ovaries; compartment-III is the anterior pituitary, which is normally responsive to the hypothalamic stimuli as well as the feedback inhibition from the ovaries; compartment-IV is a normally functioning hypothalamus integrated with higher central nervous system (CNS) centers and environmental stimuli.

After the initial history and physical examination adequacy of the outflow tract should be assessed by digital and speculum pelvic examination. Endogenous estrogen levels are assessed by observing whether the endometrium will be shed in response to a progestational challenge. Inadequate estrogen prevents the development of sufficient endometrium to be shed even when an abrupt withdrawal of a progestin is experienced. Medroxyprogesterone acetate, 10 mg PO OD ×5 days, followed by bleeding (within 7 days) is indicative of adequate estrogen but inadequate progestin effect implying anovulation (lack of progestin producing corpus luteum) as the cause of the amenorrhea.

The midcycle LH surge induces ovulation and converts the mature follicle into the corpus luteum, which produces progesterone during the second half of the 28-day cycle. If pregnancy is not achieved then there is no human chorionic gonadotropin (HCG) to provide a gonadotrophic stimulus

① Intact Comp I
② Prog challenge

PrL >20 abnl

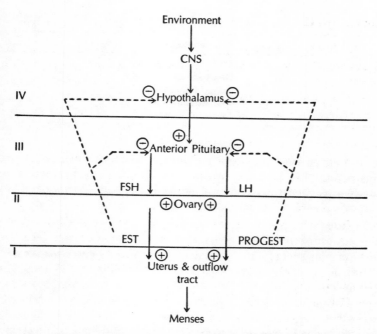

**Figure 5-1.** Compartments of the female genitourinary tract.

when LH production in the anterior pituitary declines, thus the corpus luteum undergoes involution, progesterone production falls, and the estrogen-primed endometrium is sloughed. By obtaining a menstrual period after exposure to a progestin, one has mimicked the second 14 days of a normal ovulatory cycle.

The serum prolactin (PRL) level should be measured. A level in excess of 20 mcg/liter is abnormal and by itself warrants further investigation. PRL is one of the hormones most commonly produced by a neoplastic pituitary lesion (> 50% of pituitary microadenomas). Galactorrhea is suggestive clinical evidence of hyperprolactinemia, a state that is well recognized as a potential cause of infertility. PRL excess is responsible for up to 20% of secondary amenorrhea by decreasing gonadotropin production or by de-

PRL excess → 20% of 2° amenorrhea

**TABLE 5-2. CAUSES OF HYPERPROLACTINEMIA**

| Primary | Secondary |
|---|---|
| Pituitary microadenoma | Phenothiasine drugs |
| Idiopathic | Methyldopa |
| | ↑ Estrogen excess |
| | Hepatic cirrhosis |
| | Hypothyroidism |

creasing ovarian sensitivity to the gonadotropins or both. Demonstration of a normal serum PRL, in the absence of galactorrhea, in a patient who experiences a normal progestin withdrawal bleed clinically rules out the diagnosis of hyperprolactinemia (Table 5-2).

In cases with persistent amenorrhea the next step is the provision of exogenous estrogen (2.5 mg conjugated estrogen PO OD ×21 days to prepare the endometrium for the progestin (10 mg medroxyprogesterone acetate PO OD concomitantly for the last 5 days). By providing both hormones one is testing the adequacy of the outflow tract. The lack of menses in the presence of these hormones implies discontinuity in the genitourinary tract between the endometrium and the vaginal introitus. This portion of the investigation can be omitted if there is no history of trauma or infection and the pelvic examination is within normal limits.

If the patient did not have a period in response to the progestin alone, but does in response to both estrogen and progestin, one concludes that there is an inadequacy of endogenous estrogen implicating a lesion in the ovary, pituitary, or more proximally. The next step in the investigation is to distinguish a dysfunctional pituitary from dysfunctional ovaries. This must be delayed by at least 2 weeks after the provision of exogenous estrogens because it involves the measurement of serum gonadotropin levels, which are suppressed by estrogen. The normal range for LH is between 5 and 25 IU/L (international units per litre); for FSH the normal range is 5 to 40 IU/L.

Ovarian failure causes depressed estrogen levels and elevated gonadotropin levels. Thus an LH value > 25 IU/L or an FSH value > 40 IU/L is consistent with ovarian failure, whereas abnormally low levels are suggestive of pituitary insufficiency.

LH normally spikes at the midcycle to induce ovulation, thus a high value can only be interpreted as being consistent with ovarian failure if there is no menstrual period in the 2 weeks following the determination. In clinical practice this is obviated by relying instead on the FSH determination for the diagnosis of primary ovarian failure.

An elevated FSH is indicative of sterility due to ovarian failure. A situation that will not respond to ovulatory agents (e.g., clomiphene citrate). Repetition of the test is advisable in view of the significance of the diagnosis. High serum FSH is not always synonymous with permanent ovarian failure. In *resistant ovary syndrome* the ovaries require greater than normal gonadotropin levels to provoke ovarian hormonal synthesis and function. Resistant ovary syndrome occurs in the perimenopausal age group. Primary gonadotropin-producing pituitary tumors are another rare cause of high gonadotropins without ovarian failure.

Gonadal insufficiency prior to age 35 years should prompt karyotyping studies to determine whether the patient is in fact a male pseudohermaphrodite with male gonads but female somatic sex. Ectopic male gonads are at increased risk for malignant transformation. Gonadal insufficiency over 35 years is most likely menopause and requires no further investigation.

see pg 188 ?

Hypothyroidism can be associated with menorrhagia, whereas hyperthyroidism can be associated with oligomenorrhea and amenorrhea. Both states, however, lead to impaired fertility. Thyroid investigations including free $T_4$, free $T_3$, and thyroid-stimulating hormone (TSH) levels are sufficient.

Provocative tests with luteinizing hormone releasing hormone (LHRH) intended to distinguish between hypothalamic and pituitary lesions have not proven sufficiently reliable to be recommended.

## Specific Disorders

*Compartment-I.* Infective endometritis is a rare cause of amenorrhea in North America (Fig. 5-2). The 2 principle etiologic agents are M. tuberculosis and Schistosoma. Tubercular infection is documented by culture of endometrial biopsy material or dilatation and curettage (D & C) samples.

*T.B. and Schistosoma*

**188**    OB/GYN NOTES

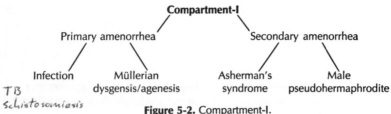

Figure 5-2. Compartment-I.

Schistosomiasis is diagnosed by visualizing the appropriate ova or parasites in the urine, stool, or endometrial tissue samples.

Asherman's syndrome is amenorrhea due to overzealous curettage which removes the regenerative basalis layer of the endometrium. Hysterosalpingography reveals multiple synechiae within the uterine cavity. Management involves lysis of adhesions with another D & C and placement of an inflated pediatric Foley catheter to prevent apposition of the uterine walls.

Müllerian dysgenesis refers to obstruction of the genitourinary system distal to the corpus uteri: cervical stenoses, vaginal canal obstructions, imperforate hymen. Müllerian agenesis (Mayer-Rokitansky-Kuster syndrome) is the second most frequent cause of primary amenorrhea. It is characterized by normal ovaries and fallopian tubes with a rudimentary uterus and only the bottom one-fifth of the vagina (urogenital sinus). Treatment consists of dilating the vaginal remnant and subsequent reconstructive surgery.

Pseudohermaphroditism is discussed in greater detail in the section on genitourinary embryology, however, any woman with inguinal hernias, unusually tall, primary amenorrhea and no uterus, or lacking body hair (undescended gonads produce insufficient androgens), should be investigated further.

**Compartment-II.** Ovarian dysgenesis (Turner's syndrome) is the most common cause of primary amenorrhea and the usual karyotype is 45-X,0 (Fig. 5-3). The common somatic stigmata of Turner's syndrome are listed:

- Low scalp
- Low ears

1° Amenorrhea          2°
① Turner's            ① stress
② Müllerian agenesis

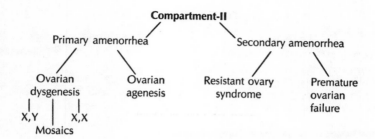

**Figure 5-3.** Compartment-II.

- High palate
- Pterygium coli
- Shield chest ⟫
- Short stature ⟫
- ↑ Carrying angle
- ↓ Fourth metacarpal
- Congenital lymphedema
- Renal anomalies
- Cardiovascular system
  Aortic coarctation
  Aortic stenosis

Ovarian dysgenesis with X,Y mosaicism has an increased risk of gonadal malignancy, whereas those with X,X mosaicism are potentially fertile but usually tend to experience premature menopause. Ovarian agenesis may present with primary amenorrhea but differs from Turner's syndrome in that it is not associated with any somatic stigmata.

Resistant ovary syndrome is a form of relative hypergonadotrophic hypogonadism that presents after the age of 30 years with oligomenorrhea. It is the result of ovarian gonadotropin insensitivity and may be associated with fertility.

***Compartment-III.*** Pituitary neoplasms very often secrete PRL, but only 33% of these will manifest clinically, e.g., galactorrhea. Pituitary hormone excess due to neoplasia often follows a predictable pattern, (PRL/GH,

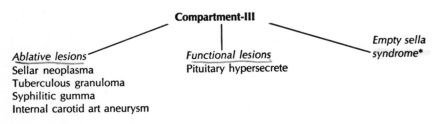

**Compartment-III**

Ablative lesions
Sellar neoplasma
Tuberculous granuloma
Syphilitic gumma
Internal carotid art aneurysm

Functional lesions
Pituitary hypersecrete

Empty sella
syndrome*

*66% of cases exhibit normal pituitary function.

**Figure 5-4.** Compartment-III.

ACTH, TSH/LH/FSH); likewise obliterative lesions lead to decreased production in a sequential pattern, (GH, FSH/LH, TSH, ACTH) (Fig. 5-4).

The *empty sella syndrome* results from congenital absence of the sellar dural diaphragm permitting extension of the subarachnoid space into the sella with resultant pituitary compression. One third of these individuals have hypogonadotrophic hypogonadism, the remainder demonstrate normal pituitary function, otherwise this is a benign condition.

*Compartment-IV.* Stress, whether physical or emotional, is the single most common cause for secondary amenorrhea. It is likely the expression of an inhibitory influence of higher CNS centers on the hypothalamus (Fig. 5-5).

If a woman is 15% or more below her ideal body weight she is likely to become amenorrheic. This is seen most commonly in the clinical settings of

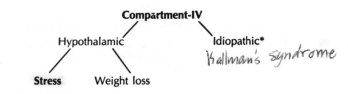

**Compartment-IV**

Hypothalamic

Idiopathic*
Kallman's syndrome

Stress    Weight loss

*Associated with anosmia.

**Figure 5-5.** Compartment-IV.

fad diets and anorexia nervosa. The mechanism through which underweight women are rendered reversibly infertile is unclear.

Amenorrhea in association with anosmia is the female counterpart to Kallmann's syndrome characterized by: primary amenorrhea, infantile genitalia, and a normal karyotype. The gonadotropin levels are low and the patient can have ovulation induced with human menopausal gonadotrophins (HMG), FSH-like activity but not with estrogen analogues, e.g., clomiphene.

## FERTILITY

Infertility is defined as the inability of a heterosexual couple to conceive after 1 year of onset of sexual relations in the absence of any form of birth control. This definition is based on certain empiric statistical observations: (1) the average time to conception for married couples is 6 months, (2) 80% of such couples conceive in 1 year, and (3) 90% have conceived within 2 years. The greater the time interval between onset of sexual relations and clinical presentation the greater the chance that the couple is infertile. One should not infer, however, that the investigations should be rigidly delayed for 2 years. Infertility can be arbitrarily classified as either primary infertility (infertility without prior pregnancy) or secondary infertility (infertility occurring after one or more pregnancies).

*Etiology and Investigations.* Infertility is the result of genitourinary or psychologic pathology within one of the sex partners of dysfunctional intercourse. The overall problem is one with which the couple must deal together regardless of the actual site of the anatomic pathology. In addition to psychologic problems and dysfunctional intercourse impairment of the following organic processes may be responsible for infertility:

| Men | Women |
|---|---|
| Spermatogenesis | Ovulation |
| Seminal fluid synthesis | Fallopian tube patency |
| Gonadal ductal system | Endometrium |
| Ejaculation | Cervical mucous |

BBT T 0.5° @ ovulation

The initial investigations of an infertile couple includes significant historical data (e.g., mumps orchitis, salpingitis) and physical examination with attention to the secondary sexual traits (see Tanner's classifications). Basic hematologic and biochemistry bloodwork can be supplemented by specific endocrine tests as indicated.

Spermatogenesis is an ongoing process throughout postpubertal life, whereas in women the majority gametogenesis occurs prenatally. Only one ovum progresses through the final meiotic division during each menstrual cycle. Thus in the adult woman oogenetic disturbances as cause of infertility are infrequent. Conversely the actual extrusion of the female gamete from the ovary (ovulation, a process without male counterpart) can be compromised. Establishing the occurrence of ovulation is discussed in detail in the section discussing ovulatory dysfunctional uterine bleeding (DUB). In review, the six lines of circumstantial evidence of ovulation are: (1) history of periodic molimina, (2) appropriate changes in vaginal cytology, (3) changes in cervical mucous viscosity and ferning characteristics, (4) a secretory pattern histologically on endometrial biopsy performed during the second half of the menstrual cycle; (5) biphasic basal body temperature (BBT) with an approximate 0.5°C rise after ovulation, and (6) plasma hormone assays (see chart in DUB section). The only definitive evidence of ovulation is pregnancy.

Fallopian tube obstruction is the single most common cause of infertility in women. In the recent past there has been a definite increase in this problem that parallels the rising incidence of salpingitis. Acquired postinflammatory cicatrization is far more common than congenital tubal obstruction. Tubal integrity and patency can be established by a number of methods. Both hysterosalpingography and laparoscopy with intrauterine dye administration are useful. The former is a procedure in which radiopaque dye is injected into the cavity of the uterine corpus via the cervix. Tubal patency is established if there is intraperitoneal "spillage" of the contrast material seen on abdominal x-ray. This procedure may have therapeutic effect in that pregnancy is noted to follow hysterosalpingography more frequently than chance alone would dictate. Laparoscopy is based on a similar principle, however, a general anesthetic is required and visualization of the intraperitoneal "spillage" is accomplished by insertion of laparoscope. Laparoscopy is particularly useful for visualization of extratubal pathology that may be missed by hysterosalpingography.

Uterine pathology may be anatomic or functional. A grossly myomatous uterus may distort the intrauterine cavity, preventing sustained nidation of the conceptus. Conversely hormonal imbalances (which may in fact be manifestations of primary pathology elsewhere) may result in an atrophic endometrium that cannot nourish the conceptus adequately. Hysterosalpingogram will document the former and endometrial biopsy is appropriate when the latter is suspect. Pelvic examination under anesthesia (EUA) is helpful in defining gross anatomic pathology of either the uterus or the adnexae when the patient cannot tolerate pelvic examination while conscious.

Cervical mucous under the influence of progestins becomes thick and ✓ viscid. If there is progestin excess (relative to estrogen) the cervical mucous may act as an effective physical barrier to sperm penetration. Agglutinating and immobilizing antisperm antibodies within the cervical mucous may be a rare cause of infertility. These factors, taken together are occasionally referred to as "cervical mucous hostility."

Semen analysis assesses both spermatogenesis and seminal fluid adequacy. Normal values are as follows:

**Spermatogenesis**

| | |
|---|---|
| Sperm count | $>60 \times 10^9/L$ |
| Motility (fractional) | $>60\%$ @ 1 hr |
| Morphology | $<20\%$ malformed |

**Seminal Fluid**

| | |
|---|---|
| Volume | 2–5 ml |
| Fructose content | $>200$ g/L |
| pH | 7.40 |
| White blood cells | None |

Testicular biopsy gives further information regarding spermatogenesis and indirect evidence of the disruption of gonadal ductal integrity (e.g., cystic fibrosis). Azoospermic seminal fluid with normal seminiferous tubule histology on biopsy is suggestive of gonadal ductal discontinuity.

**194**     OB/GYN NOTES

Ejaculatory dysfunction is usually transient and situational but may be due to serious organic pathology. A full discussion of the multidisciplinary approach to this problem can be found elsewhere. Disorders ranging from premature ejaculation to hypospadias may be responsible for limiting ejaculatory efficiency and therefore infertility.

An assessment of the efficacy of coital technique can be obtained by history and more objectively by performing a **postcoital test.** The latter consists of examining posterior forniceal fluid samples within an hour of coitus to ascertain whether sperm are present.

*Therapeutic Interventions.* Induction of either ovulation or spermatogenesis may be attempted by means of human menopausal gonadotropins (HMG), FSH-like activity, HCG, LH-like activity, and a nonsteroidal estrogen analogue, clomiphene citrate. Bromocriptine, a dopamine agonist, is useful for documented cases of idiopathic hyperprolactinemia. Fallopian tube, anatomic uterine, and male gonadal ductal pathology is usually addressed surgically.

For cervical mucous antisperm antibodies, temporary abstinence is advised to decrease the amount of antibody formed through repeat antigen exposure. Intermittent abstinence has only limited success.

A variety of procedures and techniques are available for those who wish to have children of their own despite proven lesions rendering one partner infertile. These include: artificial insemination homologous (**AIH**), i.e., the usual male sex partner is the sperm donor; artificial insemination donor (**AID**), i.e., an anonymous male is the sperm donor; **in vitro fertilization** (fertilization of ovum by sperm occurs within laboratory apparatus) and surrogate motherhood. Adoption as a means of fulfilling parental desire is greatly limited by the rising rate of induced abortions.


## DYSFUNCTIONAL UTERINE BLEEDING

Dysfunctional uterine bleeding is the gynecologic term for abnormal periods. Normal menses are defined as a **bloody vaginal discharge** that is **spontaneous and periodic** and represents **postovulatory endometrial**

24 - 32 d
3 - 7 d
< 80 ml (avg 33 ml)

**shedding.** Clinically a normal period is defined by (1) **interval,** 24 to 32 days (time between periods); (2) **duration,** 3 to 7 days; and (3) **volume,** < 80 ml (the average is ~33 ml, 80% of which is discharged during the first  ✗ 2 days).

Any bloody vaginal discharge whose interval, duration, or frequency is at odds with the normals for a given patient, excluding any obvious cause, represents DUB. The initial step in diagnosis is to ensure that perineal blood loss is truly of uterine origin. Patient age and the pattern of blood loss are important historical features that aid diagnosis.

✓ Three gross distinctions can be made with respect to patient age: perimenarchal (anovulatory cycles common); childbearing age (vaginal bleeding is usually related either to conception or contraception); and perimenopausal age (local anatomic pathology common).

There exist a number of increasingly obsolete terms used to describe the various patterns of vaginal bleeding.

| | | |
|---|---|---|
| *Oligomenorrhea*<br>Interval > 40 days | vs. | *Polymenorrhea*<br>Interval < 21 days |
| *Hypomenorrhea*<br>↓ Volume +/−<br>↓ duration | vs. | *Hypermenorrhea*<br>↑ Volume +/−<br>↑ duration |
| *Metrorrhagia*<br>Variable intervals | vs. | *Menometrorrhagia*<br>Variable interval and<br>↑ Volume +/− ↑ duration |
| *Intermenstrual*<br>Occurring between<br>otherwise normal periods | vs. | *Postmenopausal*<br>Occurring after the menopause |

These terms often lead to confusion, therefore it is suggested that the pattern of bleeding be described by the interval, duration, and volume as reported by the patient.

The past medical history may yield significant diagnostic information (e.g., thyroid dysfunction, bleeding disorder).

It is important to determine whether DUB was associated with an

*Anovulatory cycles can cause
* abnl periods

Estrogen          Progestins
196    OB/GYN NOTES   acidophilic cells    basophilic
       high  KPI            low KPI

ovulatory or anovulatory period. Anovulatory cycles can cause abnormal periods. Circumstantial evidence that supports the occurrence of ovulation takes several forms: (1) historical reports of mastalgia, transient weight gain, cramping, and predictable periodicity; (2) estrogen-induced cervical mucous characteristics, ie. decreased viscosity (*spinnbarkeit*) and prominent "ferning" on drying (recall that the midcycle LH surge held responsible for ovulation is likely the result of positive feedback of rapidly rising estrogen levels on the pituitary); (3) biphasic BBT, with progestin mediated temperature elevation (~0.5°C) during the latter half of the cycle; (4) vaginal cytology (preovulatory estrogen results in prominence of acidophilic cells with high karyopyknotic index (KPI), whereas postovulatory progestins result in the prominence of basophilic cells with low KPI); (5) endometrial biopsy during second half of the menstrual cycle that reveals a progestin supported secretory pattern; and (6) plasma hormone assays (Fig. 5-6). Parenthetically, the only definitive proof of ovulation is pregnancy.

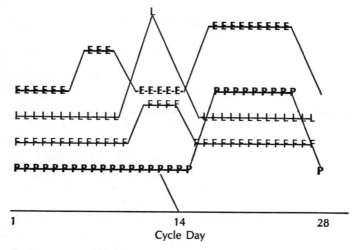

E, estrogen; F, follicle-stimulating hormone; L, luteinizing hormone; P, progesterone.

**Figure 5-6.** Normal cyclic hormonal variations.

*BBT, 5 c° Progestin mediated.*

The potential causes of DUB are reviewed in three major groupings: (1) DUB occurring with anovulatory cycles, (2) with ovulatory cycles, and (3) during pregnancy.

## DUB Associated With Anovulation

Anovulatory cycles are usually associated with polymenorrhea or hypermenorrhagia. Anovulatory DUB is usually transient and self-limited, e.g., perimenarchal. Anovulation is most often the result of an endocrine imbalance. Dysfunction of the hypothalamic–pituitary–ovarian (H–P–O) system can be broken down into that due to central (CNS, hypothalamus, pituitary), intermediate (the influence of other endocrine glands on the H–P–O axis), or peripheral (ovaries) causes.

Of the central causes by far the most common is psychogenic stress. The mechanism through which stress affects menstrual discharge is not known.

One of the key changes associated with puberty is the alteration of hypothalamic sensitivity to estrogen-induced negative feedback. At puberty hypothalamic estrogen sensitivity falls thus higher estrogen levels (sufficient to promote development of secondary sexual characteristics) are required to inhibit LHRH secretion to any given degree. If the hypothalamus retains its prepubertal estrogen sensitivity, estrogen could not mediate the midcycle LH surge triggering ovulation.

Oral contraceptive pills (OCPs) are intended to cause anovulatory cycles, thus preventing the possibility of pregnancy. OCP's usually cause hypomenorrhea because of the predominance of the progestogenic component in most formulations. Relative estrogen inadequacy can lead to "breakthrough" bleeding (endometrial basalis layer hemorrhage) or prolonged amenorrhea (sufficient endometrial spongiosa to prevent basalis hemorrhage but insufficient to cause endometrial sloughing). OCP's with relative estrogen excess can cause prolonged amenorrhea followed by hypermenorrhagia (fragile overproliferated endometrium can no longer be adequately vascularized and sloughs spontaneously).

Other endocrine glands that can influence endometrial shedding include the thyroid and the adrenals. Adrenocortical hypersecretion does not usually result in anovulation until the primary lesion is clinically apparent. Hypothy-

Testosterone → estradiol
Androstenedione → estrone

(?) see page 187

roidism can cause oligomenorrhea whereas hyperthyroidism causes hypermenorrhagia.

Variations in body weight also affect menstrual blood loss. Significantly underweight patients can have hypomenorrhea or amenorrhea. The pathophysiology is not understood. Individuals that are morbidly obese have tonically elevated estrogen levels and therefore menometrorrhagia. The peripheral (white) adipose tissue acts to convert testosterone (from female gonads) and androstenedione (from adrenals) to estradiol and estrone, respectively.

Polycystic ovarian disease (PCOD) or Stein-Leventhal syndrome is another entity associated with abnormal uterine bleeding and anovulatory cycles. The primary lesion has not been defined. It may represent an anomalous central insensitivity to estrogen positive feedback or a primary ovarian disorder in which the follicle fails to develop fully thus synthesizing inadequate quantities of estrogen to trigger the midcycle LH surge.

Clinically the constellation of signs and symptoms may include any or all of the following: obesity, hirsuitism, cushingoid appearance, galactorrhea, and DUB. Hormonal aberrations have been observed that may account for some of these changes but it is unclear, as stated above, which of these represents the inciting factor. Adrenocortical overactivity produces increased amounts of androstenedione, the excess peripheral adipose tissue promotes conversion of androstenedione to estrone. LH, in turn, remains tonically elevated rather than exhibiting its usual marked fluctuation and midcycle surge. FSH for unexplained reasons remains normal or suppressed. Prolactin conversely is normal or elevated. Not surprisingly the endometrium is hyperplastic (initially cystic, then adenomatous) due to the continuous unopposed estrone. PCOD increases the risk of adenocarcinoma of the uterine corpus.

Treatment for this entity addresses the presenting complaint. If the chief problem is hirsuitism, then OCPs are prescribed to provide a supply of female sex steroid and to inhibit gonadotropin secretion (LH excess may promote gonadal testosterone synthesis). If DUB is the reason for presentation then cyclic progestins will ensure predictable withdrawal bleeds. Infertility can be addressed by use of the central estrogen antagonist clomiphene citrate.

Peripheral causes of DUB include functional ovarian neoplasms. The granulosa cell tumor can cause menometrorrhagia or precocious puberty with premature menarche. Primary ovarian insufficiency, whether it be congenital (Turner's syndrome) or acquired (menopausal) leads to hypomenorrhea or amenorrhea. Functional cysts, such as persistent corpus luteum, may also lead to amenorrhea.

## DUB Associated With Ovulation

Follicular insufficiency, luteal insufficiency and irregular endometrial shedding, may be clinically indistinguishable in patients complaining of more frequent periods (polymenorrhea). One may be able to elicit a history of predictable regularity in patients with follicular insufficiency. Accurate BBT recordings can aid in diagnosis. Both follicular and luteal insufficiency give biphasic recordings but follicular insufficiency is characterized by shortening of the first (lower temperature) phase of the BBT to < 10 days; whereas luteal insufficiency is characterized by shortening of the second (higher temperature) phase of the BBT recording to < 10 d patients with luteal insufficiency may also have a history of repeat first trimester spontaneous abortions. Follicular insufficiency is treated with estrogen supplementation during the follicular phase of the cycle to ensure 13 days of endometrial proliferation; luteal insufficiency is treated with progesterone supplementation during the luteal phase of the cycle to ensure a 13-day secretory phase.

Irregular endometrial shedding is due to progesterone excess. The diagnosis is established by endometrial biopsy on the fifth day of the cycle, which exhibits the anomalous persistence of a secretory endometrium. Low-dose estrogenic supplementation started on the first day of the cycle is indicated.

Bleeding diatheses, whether congenital (e.g., von Willebrand's disease, autosomal dominant) or acquired (idiopathic thrombocytopenic purpura) can clearly result in excessive endometrial blood loss. Regularity of the menses is usually retained but they are heavier than normal (i.e., increased volume).

Iatrogenic DUB may result from anticoagulant therapy or from intrauterine devices (IUDs). The hypermenorrhagia associated with IUD's is usually self-limited after several cycles.

Chronic renal failure is usually associated with amenorrhea, oligomenorrhea, or metrorrhagia, whereas effective dialytic therapy often leads to menorrhagia. Interestingly, successful transplantation of a functional renal allograft results in normalization of the process in about 60% of cases.

Anatomic lesions that can disturb menses can be addressed systematically as lesions involving the uterine cervix, the uterine corpus, or the adnexae.

Cervical polyps present with light posttraumatic (postcoital, after straining at stool, or after douche), or intermenstrual hemorrhage. A biopsy of the lesion is required to ensure that it is not a prolapsed submucosal myoma or a malignancy. Ectropion may cause similar clinical presentation. Cervical eversion of friable endocervical epithelium should also be biopsied to rule out malignancy. Carcinoma of the cervix also gives rise to posttraumatic and intermenstrual bleeding, with or without, a visible lesion. Exfoliative cytology, colposcopy, and directed biopsy are indicated as discussed elsewhere in the notes.

Endometrial polyps are clinically indistinguishable from cervical polyps. The bleeding results from superficial ulceration. Cramping may occur if the polyp infarcts and sloughs. Chronic endometritis is not a common occurrence and should prompt one to consider the possibility of smoldering upper tract disease, e.g., hydrosalpinx or pyosalpinx, salpingitis, retained IUD or products of conception. Acute endometritis can be seen as part of the cervicitis and salpingitis of pelvic inflammatory disease (PID) or localized acute infections of endometrial tissues overlying submucous myomas or polyps. In addition to the previously mentioned inflammatory processes, GU neoplastia can cause DUB. These include malignancies, such as uterine adenocarcinoma and sarcoma, as well as benign entities such as myomas. Myomas are so common, that the diagnosis of myoma as cause of DUB can only be made after other causes have been ruled out. Note also that only submucous or interstitial myomas are capable of causing menstrual irregularity. Myoma should not be proposed as the cause of postmenopausal DUB because it is almost exclusively limited to the childbearing years. Uterine bleeding occurring after the menopause is highly suggestive of malignancy.

The most common adnexal pathology likely to alter menstrual function

*only submucous or interstitial myomas are capable of causing menstrual irregularity. (Not subserousal myoma)*

is salpingitis, but carcinoma of the tube or ovary should also be considered. Tubal carcinoma, although exceedingly rare, presents with a characteristic serosanguinous discharge (hydrosalpinx perfluens) due to intratubal epithelial ulceration.

## DUB Associated With Pregnancy

Most of these entities have been discussed in other sections. Uterine bleeding during pregnancy is usually problematic in the initial or final trimesters as well as in the immediate postpartum period.

Problems that arise in the first trimester include spontaneous abortion and ectopic pregnancy. Gestational trophoblastic disease (hydatidiform mole) also presents at this time and is discussed in a separate section. Third-trimester problems and post-partum hemorrhage are covered in the section on vaginal bleeding in pregnancy. The most common causes of PPH are uterine atony, retained placenta, uterine laceration, and bleeding diatheses.

*Treatment.* The goals of therapy are (1) to maintain hemodynamic stability; (2) secure hemostasis; and (3) prevent recurrence. The first two goals involve acute resuscitative measures (intravenous crystalloid with urine output or central venous pressure monitoring, or both, in addition to either suction or "chemical" curettage. Curettage should not be undertaken if one has strong reason to believe that the patient is pregnant or has a bleeding diathesis. The choice of medical or surgical approach is based on the acuteness, frequency, and severity of the problem. If the patient is relatively stable, then one can take a more conservative, medical approach to the problem. Chemical curettage may be accomplished by giving progesterone, 100 to 200 mg IM, which may be repeated in 2 to 4 hours followed by medroxyprogesterone acetate, 10 to 20 mg PO OD for 10 days. An alternate approach is to administer large doses of combination OCPs, tapering the dosage over 14 to 21 days. Endometrial slouching usually occurs within 2 to 3 days of hormonal (progestin) withdrawal.

Current controversy centers around the efficacy of intravenous estrogen in the acute situation. Proponents claim that the estrogen acutely increases the availability of blood coagulation factors thus promoting hemostasis. Detractors state that uterine hemostasis is primarily dependent on kinking of intramural vasculature by the contracted myometrium, a process in which estrogen plays no significant role.

The regularization of menstrual blood loss can be achieved with either OCPs or intermittent short courses of progestin therapy. The patient should be informed that the latter does not constitute an effective mode of contraception.

## DYSMENORRHEA

Painful menstruation or dysmenorrhea is one of the most common gynecologic complaints with up to 10% of women experiencing pain of sufficient intensity to cause incapacity for 1 to 3 days per month. Dysmenorrhea is arbitrarily divided into two entities to facilitate diagnosis. **Primary dysmenorrhea** occurs in the absence of detectable pelvic pathology, whereas **secondary dysmenorrhea** is associated with another gynecologic disorder (see pelvic pain section).

Primary dysmenorrhea manifests as a colicky suprapubic discomfort that may radiate to the sacrum or the medial aspect of the thighs. Discomfort usually commences synchronously with menstrual flow and subsides within hours (may persist for days). Nonspecific gastrointestinal (nausea, vomiting, diarrhea) and central nervous system (headache, dizziness) complaints often accompany dysmenorrhea. Primary dysmenorrhea usually begins several months or even years after menarche. The pain is attributed to excessive prostaglandin-induced (primarily $PGF_{2\alpha}$) myometrial contraction. Local uterine production of prostaglandins is enhanced by progesterone. It has been suggested that the occurrence of ovulation and luteal phase is prerequisite for dysmenorrhea. Perimenarchal anovulatory menstrual cycles not be associated with dysmenorrhea. The problem often abates progressively with age or after pregnancy for unknown reasons.

Primary dysmenorrhea has not been associated with hormonal imbalance.

Secondary dysmenorrhea is discussed in the section on pelvic pain and elsewhere under the headings of the specific disorders involved. Any form of dysmenorrhea that begins for the first time after pregnancy or after 20 years of age must be highly suspect as a form of secondary dysmenorrhea.

*NSAIDs impair hemostasis + exacerbate Na/H₂O retention by interfering c prostaglandins at platelets + nephron.*

Although the pain of dysmenorrhea is real, the interpretation of its severity is strongly influenced by learned behavior. The same degree of discomfort may go unnoticed in one patient and cause monthly invalidism in another. This factor cannot be ignored in the management of primary dysmenorrhea.

Once pelvic pathology has been ruled out, mild dysmenorrhea may be managed with symptomatic measures (e.g., local heat) and reeducation. For more severe pain the nonsteroidal anti-inflammatory drugs (NSAIDs) have been hailed as specific therapy because of their action as prostaglandin synthetase inhibitors:

## NSAIDs

| | |
|---|---|
| ASA | 650 mg PO q4-6h |
| Mefenamic acid | 500 mg PO QID |
| Naproxen | 500 mg PO BID |
| Indomethacin | 25–50 mg PO T-QID |
| Ibuprofen | 400–800 mg PO QID |

Acetaminophen may cause less GI upset but constitutes only symptomatic (analgesic therapy). NSAID's can impair hemostasis and exacerbate $NA^+/H_2O$ retention by interfering with prostaglandin function at the platelets and nephron, respectively.

Dysmenorrhea refractory to the prostaglandin synthetase inhibitors may be treated with OCPs to induce anovulatory cycles. If medical management is unsuccessful, then presacral neurotomy may be performed as a last resort, usually with good relief.

## PREMENSTRUAL TENSION SYNDROME

*∅ dysmenorrhea assoc c ovulatory cycles ∅ hormonal imbalance*

Premenstrual tension (PMT) syndrome consists of regular cyclic mastodynia, peripheral edema (weight gain, > 2 kg), headache, and variable emotional lability during the 4 to 10 days preceding menstrual flow. Dys- *+* menorrhea, once menstrual flow commences, is distinctly unusual. PMT is usually associated with ovulatory cycles and as yet no hormonal imbalance has been causally associated with this problem. The etiology is unknown but

*= mastodynia =*

environmental stress and secondary hyperaldosteronism (perhaps mediated by an unusually sensitive sympathetic nervous system) have been invoked, despite being unable to document the expected fluid/ electrolyte imbalance of hyperaldosteronism. As for primary dysmenorrhea the role of psychologic factors cannot be ignored.

Spironolactone or thiazide diuretics may be suggested especially if edema is particularly troublesome. Pyridoxine (vitamin $B_6$ in total daily doses of up to 1.0 g PO) and anxiolytic medications have also been used. OCPs are variably effective, occasionally exacerbating the problem. Severe forms of emotional lability associated with this disorder resemble psychotic behavior and may warrant psychiatric referral.

# 6

# Birth Control

## ORAL CONTRACEPTIVE PILL

The development of the oral contraceptive pill (OCP) in the 1960s heralded the era of reliable, reversible reproductive control (Table 6-1). OCPs are the most effective reversible method of contraception, the failure rate being ~0.3 in 100,000.

The combination OCP acts by supplying pharmacologic levels of both ovarian sex steroids that suppress CNS neuroendocrine organs resulting in decreased gonadotropin secretion mimicking the pregnant state. Ovulatory suppression is related to the estrogen and progestin content as well as the ratio of one to the other within a given formulation.

The estrogen content of the OCP modulates the degree of endometrial sloughing at the end of each menstrual cycle. High estrogen levels result in excessive proliferation of the endometrium with spontaneous sloughing of the surface (in the absence of progestin withdrawal). Too thick to be vascularized adequately the upper layers infarct and slough. Less estrogen results in endometrial proliferation but no sloughing unless progestin withdrawal is experienced. This resembles the physiologic process. Slightly lower estrogen levels cause less than normal endometrial proliferation such that progestin withdrawal induces minimal or no sloughing (hypomenorrhea or amenorrhea). This situation is commonly achieved through the use of OCPs. Very low levels of estrogen result in an atrophic endometrium that inadequately covers the underlying myometrium and basal layer of endometrium, which may, therefore, bleed spontaneously and irregularly (so-

*Too low levels of estrogen → Atrophic myometrium leading to break through bleeding.*

**TABLE 6-1. INDICATIONS AND CONTRAINDICATIONS TO THE USE OF OCP**

| Indications | Contraindications |
|---|---|
| Contraception | Pregnancy |
| Dysmenorrhea | ✗ Thromboembolic disease[a] (TED) |
| Menorrhagia | Acute liver disease |
| Dysfunctional uterine bleeding[a] | Estrogen-dependent neoplasia |
| ✗ Chronic cystic mastitis (recurrent breast lumps) | ✗ Undiagnosed abnormal vaginal bleeding |
| Acne | ✗ Ocular lesions |

[a]Certain forms of DUB only—see section on DUB.

*Prog predominates*

called **breakthrough bleeding**). Although the progestational effect always predominates with respect to reproductive tract end organs (thin endometrium, thick cervical mucous) the estrogen is said to "stabilize" the endometrium by preventing total atrophy with breakthrough bleeding.

The thinning of the endometrium and the thickening of the cervical mucous, as well as a lowering of the vaginal pH (sperm thrive best in alkaline medium), all contribute to the overall contraceptive effect of the OCP. A thin endometrium is unsuitable for nidation even if conception does occur and thick cervical mucous impedes sperm access.

Presently all OCPs available on the market are combinations of orally active estrogens and 19-nortestosterone derivatives that exhibit progestational effects. The estrogenic component is either ethinyl estradiol (EE) or 3-methylether-EE (also known as mestranol) and both retain oral efficacy. The 19-nortestosterones, as the name implies are modified androgenic hormones but their metabolites also manifest estrogenic effects.

The relative potencies of the currently available synthetic sex steroids listed in descending order are: (1) **estrogenic** ethinyl estradiol, mestranol; (2) **progestational,** norgestrel, ethynodiol diacetate, levonorgestrel, norethynodrel, norethindrone acetate, norethindrone; (3) **androgenic,** norgestrel, norethindrone, norethindrone acetate, ethynodiol diacetate, norethynodrel.

In addition to the possible side effects of OCPs, there are a number of conditions that are commonly exacerbated and others commonly improved by OCPs.

| OCP Liabilities | OCP Benefits |
|---|---|
| ↑ Hypertension | ↓ Dysmenorrhea |
| ↑ Impairment of glucose homeo- stasis | ↓ Anemia due to menstrual blood loss |
| ↑ Frequency of epileptic seizures | ↓ Risk of endometrial cancer |
| Worsening of migraines | ↓ Incidence of benign breast disease ovarian cysts/cancer ectopic pregnancy |

Table 6-2 lists the various trade preparations, indicating the combination of estrogen and progestin present in each formulation.

## OCP Side Effects

There are many possible side effects associated with combination OCPs. Most are minor or self-limited, but they can be severe enough to warrant discontinuation. Side effects are listed under three headings: (1) female reproductive tract side effects, (2) general metabolic side effects, and (3) other organ system side effects.

*Female Reproductive Tract Side Effects.* Initially it was felt that "postpill" amenorrhea was a distinct clinical entity consisting of secondary amenorrhea after prolonged use of OCPs due to a poorly delineated form of hypothalamic suppression. Presently, however, it is felt to have been a statistical byproduct of more zealous follow-up than for the general population. The estrogenic component of the OCP is held responsible for increased breast tenderness and a decrease in the quantity and quality of breastmilk but the OCP has not been proven to induce malignant breast neoplasia in humans. Indeed the progestin is credited with decreasing the incidence of benign breast lesions. Estrogen may promote enlargement of leiomyomas. The relative predominance of the progestin over estrogen with respect to the reproductive tract often results in hypomenorrhea. There is an increased frequency of abnormal cervical cytology but no increase in malignant or

Polypoid Adenomatous hyperpl.
of the endocx is an effect
of estrogen.

208

## TABLE 6-2. ORAL CONTRACEPTIVE PILL FORMULATIONS

| Drug | Estrogen | Amount (mcg) | Progestin | Amount (mg) |
|---|---|---|---|---|
| Ovulen | Mestranol | 100 | ED | 1.0 |
| Enovid-E | Mestranol | 100 | Norethynodrel | 2.5 |
| Ortho-Novum 2 mg | Mestranol | 100 | Norethindrone | 2.0 |
| Norinyl 2 mg | Mestranol | 100 | Norethindrone | 2.0 |
| Ortho-Novum 1/80 | Mestranol | 80 | Norethindrone | 1.0 |
| Norinyl 1+80 | Mestranol | 80 | Norethindrone | 1.0 |
| Enovid 5 mg | Mestranol | 75 | Norethyndrel | 5.0 |
| Demulen | EE | 50 | ED | 1.0 |
| Ovral | EE | 50 | Norgestrel | 0.5 |
| Norlestrin 2.5/50 | EE | 50 | NA | 2.5 |
| Norlestrin 1/50 | EE | 50 | NA | 1.0 |
| Ovcon-50 | EE | 50 | Norethindrone | 1.0 |
| Norinyl 1+50 | Mestranol | 50 | Norethindrone | 1.0 |
| Ortho-Novum 1/50 | Mestranol | 50 | Norethindrone | 1.0 |
| Demulen 1/35 | EE | 35 | ED | 1.0 |
| Norinyl 1+35 | EE | 35 | Norethindrone | 1.0 |
| Ortho-Novum 1/35 | EE | 35 | Norethindrone | 1.0 |
| Ortho-Novum 10/11 | EE | 35 | Norethindrone | 0.5 |
| followed by | EE | 35 | Norethindrone | 1.0 |
| Triphasil | EE | 30 | Norgestrel | 0.05 |
| ×6 days | | | | |
| followed by | EE | 40 | Norgestrel | 0.075 |
| ×5 days | | | | |
| followed by | EE | 30 | Norgestrel | 0.125 |
| ×10 days | | | | |
| Brevicon | EE | 35 | Norethindrone | 0.5 |
| Modicon | EE | 35 | Norethindrone | 0.5 |
| Ovcon-35 | EE | 35 | Norethindrone | 0.4 |
| Lo/Ovral | EE | 30 | Norgestrel | 0.3 |
| Loestrin 1.5/30 | EE | 30 | NA | 1.5 |
| Nordette | EE | 30 | Levonorgestrel | 0.15 |
| Loestrin 1/20 | EE | 20 | NA | 1.0 |
| Ovrette | nil | | Norgestrel | 0.075 |
| Nor-Q.D. | nil | | Norethindrone | 0.35 |
| Micronor | nil | | Norethindrone | 0.35 |

ED, ethyniodial diacetate; EE, ethinyl estradiol; NA, norethinodrone acetate.

premalignant cervical lesions. Polypoidal adenomatous hyperplasia of the endocervix is promoted (estrogen effect), but this is not a premalignant lesion. Within the vagina there is an alteration in the normal bacterial flora (estrogen) effect, which may promote vaginal candidosis. The increased incidence of other sexually transmitted diseases cannot, however, be attributed directly to an OCP effect.

### General Metabolic Side Effects

*Protein Metabolism.* Estrogens, being anabolic steroids, are capable of increasing protein synthesis. Clinically significant proteins affected in this manner include the blood coagulation factors (BCF) and angiotensinogen, both members of the alpha-2 globulins. Angiotensinogen is converted to angiotensin-II by renin secreted from the kidney and pulmonary angiotension converting enzyme. Angiotensin-II promotes fluid retention and vasoconstriction resulting in increased blood pressure. The elevation in serum levels of BCFs as well as an increased propensity of platelets to aggregate are thought to underlie the heightened risk of thromboembolic disease (TED) associated with OCP use. TED may manifest at many sites in the vasculature: cerebral circulation, retina, heart, extremities (with possible pulmonary embolism), and mesenteric system. Estrogen is also responsible for the wholesale increase in the levels of serum carrier proteins. The increase in thyroid binding globulin (TBG) and cortisol binding globulin (CBG) results in increases in the commonly used assays for measuring total thyroid hormone and cortisol. In fact, the free fraction of hormone changes only minimally. Although sex hormone binding globulin (SHBG) levels rise, testosterone production does not keep pace, therefore the "free" (active) fraction actually declines. This may be responsible for the decrease in libido observed in some patients using OCPs. The increase in alpha-2 globulins is also responsible for erythrocyte sedimentation rate (ESR) elevations seen in (pregnancy and) OCP users.    ESR ↑

*Carbohydrate Metabolism.* There is a notable increase in peripheral insulin resistance. Taken together with the small but real increase in free cortisol levels glucose tolerance becomes impaired. Most individuals have sufficient insulin reserve to prevent clinical presentation. Alterations in glucose tolerance due to OCPs usually revert to normal when they are discontinued.

*Lipid Metabolism.* Increased insulin levels (due to insulin resistance) may have a spillover effect on hepatic lipid synthesis leading to an increase in triglyceride and phospholipid synthesis. There may also be a decrease in adipose tissue triglyceride uptake due to insulin mediated inhibition of lipoprotein lipase activity. Both mechanisms act to elevate serum lipid levels.

↑ serum lipids

### Other Organ System Side Effects

*Hepatobiliary System.* There is an increased incidence of hepatoma (primarily associated with mestranol-containing preparations). Histologically benign, it may, nevertheless, lead to serious hemorrhagic complications. There may also be an increase in the cholesterol fraction of bile, which may promote cholelithiasis and cholestasis.

*Neuropsychiatric.* An increased incidence of migraine, epileptic seizures, and strokes is noted. It is important to note that serious neurologic side effects, although statistically more common in OCP users than in the general population, are still quite rare.

In the central nervous system (CNS) tryptophan can be metabolized to either 5-hydroxytryptamine (5-HT) (serotonin) or nicotine adenine dinucleotide (NAD). Estrogen seems to siphon CNS tryptophan toward NAD, depleting the CNS supply of 5-HT. This has been correlated with clinical depression, which may be responsive to pyridoxine (vitamin $B_6$) therapy for as yet unknown reasons.

*Skin and Gastrointestinal System.* Chloasma occurs rarely, and if it does, it resolves slowly. The effect of an OCP on acne depends on the relative potency of the two components; estrogen promotes clearing, whereas synthetic progestins are androgenic and, therefore, worsen the skin condition.

Oral contraceptive pills can cause nausea and less commonly even

Acne: estrogen promotes clearing
Progestins (androgenic) worsens skin cond.

TABLE 6-3. DRUG INTERACTIONS

| Agents That Diminish OCP Effect | Agents Whose Effect is Altered By OCPs |
|---|---|
| Anticonvulsants | Anticonvulsants |
| Antibiotics | Anticoagulants (oral) |
| Antacids | Antihypertensives |
| Sedative/hypnotics | Sedative/hypnotics |
| | Oral hypoglycemics |
| | Folate preparations |
| | Alcohol |
| | Hypolipidemic agents |

For a more complete listing of specific interactions one may consult The Medical Letter Handbook of Drug Interactions, MA Rizack (ed), pp 42–45, 1983.

vomiting. They also promote weight gain. The initial 1 to 2 kg is estrogen-mediated fluid retention (R/A/A system), further gains are attributable to androgenic hypothalamic appetite stimulation mediated by the synthetic progestins.

## Drug Interactions
Drug interactions with OCPS are listed in Table 6-3.

*Therapeutic Principles.* Before starting steroid contraception the initial interview should be used to establish the need for contraception and the best form of contraception suitable for each particular patient taking into account such factors as the age, motivation, and sexual practices of the patient as well as those of her partner(s). Factors that may predispose to TED must also be sought. The patient should be actively encouraged to read the package insert and the physician should be available to discuss any questions that may arise. The initial physical examination should include breast, liver, and extremity examination (potential source of thromboembolism), as well as a pelvic examination with Pap smear and urinalysis.

Smoking, parity, and age are three significant independent risk factors that must be taken into consideration when advising a patient about the choice of contraception to be employed. Smoking raises the risk of death due to OCP use from 1.6 to 10.2 per 100,000. Similarly increasing parity and age (especially when > 35 years) increase morbidity and mortality of OCP use.

Currently it is suggested that patients started on OCPs be seen for initial follow-up at 3 months and thereafter every 12 months, (q6mo for adolescents). Follow-up examination should include (1) history to exclude newly acquired contraindications, (2) liver, breast, and pelvic examination with Pap smear, (3) urinalysis, and (4) blood pressure check.

Although it is commonly accepted that most morbidity and mortality is attributable to the estrogenic component of the combination OCP and that these problems are dose related it is becoming increasingly apparent that the synthetic progestins are at least in part responsible for some of the side effects. Combination OCPs containing 30 to 35 mcg of estrogen are no less effective in preventing pregnancy than those containing more estrogen. For this reason it is suggested that OCPs containing minimum effective levels of both estrogen (30 to 35 mcg) and progestin be the initial agent chosen. Proof of significant reductions of morbidity or mortality from use of such formulations is not yet available. Should breakthrough bleeding occur, additional estrogen in the form of ethinyl estradiol, 20 mcg PO OD, or conjugated estrogens, 2.5 mg PO OD (either for 7 days), may be helpful.

Oral contraceptive pills should be commenced on the fifth day of a normal period (note the first day of the menstrual cycle is arbitrarily defined as the first day of bleeding). This ensures that the patient is not pregnant at the start and subsequent ovulation is sufficiently far off that it should be successfully inhibited by the OCP. If this timing is strictly adhered to then one need not advise the use of an alternate mode of contraception during the first cycle of OCP use as was routinely done in the past.

Oral contraceptive pills are provided in two formats: 21 OCPs or 21 OCPs with 7 inert (or iron tablets) tablets for a total of 28 tablets. The latter format is usually reserved for those patients that are less reliable (e.g., adolescents) (Fig. 6-1).

Amenorrhea while a patient is taking the pill should always trigger an investigation for possible pregnancy. With pregnancy ruled out, amenorrhea is most suggestive of an estrogen level sufficient to prevent breakthrough bleeding but insufficient to provide endometrial material for sloughing at the end of the period. The patient may then be switched to a 50-mcg estrogen formulation.

↑ risk of T-E phenomena 2 wks pp.

*21-Day Format*

```
        26-----4  5-  ------    ------  ---25  26-----4  Cycle Day #
        1-nil--7  1******OCPs*******21  1-nil--7  Tablet #
```

*28-Day Format*

```
        26 ----- 4  5-  ------    ------  ---25  26 ----- 4  Cycle Day #
        1-plac--7  1******OCPs*******21  1-plac--7  Tablet #
```

**plac,** placebo.

**Figure 6-1.** OCP formats.

The first two postpartum weeks represent a high-risk interval for thromboembolic phenomena thus estrogen containing contraceptives should be avoided. Ovulation is physiologically delayed by a term pregnancy for about 4 to 6 weeks. If oral steroid contraception is to be undertaken it is best initiated ~3 weeks after delivery. ⊛

Although it had been previously suggested that a "rest" from OCPs was advisable at fairly regular intervals to permit the hypothalamic–pituitary–ovarian axis to reestablish normal control over the menstrual cycle there is no proof that such OCP "holidays" are necessary.

# INTRAUTERINE DEVICE

Intrauterine devices (IUDs) made of various plastics, in numerous shapes, with or without copper and progesterone, act to create an endometrial surface that is less suitable for nidation of the conceptus. Thus, in fact these devices do not prevent conception. They act to produce abortion usually within the first week after conception.

Plain IUDs without copper or progesterone are thought to induce a local sterile inflammatory process in the endometrial tissue thus rendering it less capable of sustaining nidation. The increased frequency of infectious endometritis and endosalpingitis associated with IUDs is thought to underlie the increased incidence of tubal pregnancy in these patients.

IUD's are used as a form of birth control that results from automatic, efficacious induced abortion. For many this is an acceptable form of controlling reproductive potential.

Copper is included in some devices because of its putative spermicidal effects and because it may also be capable of decreasing gonococcal viability. Should local infection occur, the device must be removed. Copper-containing devices normally require replacement every 24 to 36 months. *hypermature endometrium* Progesterone-laden devices act to thicken cervical mucous and thin the endometrial tissue. The latter effect results in decreased menstrual blood loss or even amenorrhea rather than the menorrhagia usually observed with IUD use. These devices must normally be replaced every 12 to 18 months to maintain efficacy.

## Contraindications
Contraindications to IUD use are listed in Table 6-4.

## Morbidity and Mortality
Relatively minor side effects include dysmenorrhea and menometrorrhagia, both of which are often transient. If more severe, they may lead to discontinuation of IUD use. Serious side effects include uterine perforation (more common with early postpartum insertion) and salpingitis (with an unexplained propensity for unilateral tubal involvement and a disproportionately higher incidence of actinomycotic infections). Salpingitis carries with it the risk of sterility due to intratubal or peritubal cicatrization, therefore, this method is not suggested as a primary method of contraception for nulliparous women.

In review the morbidity of IUD use is greater than that of OCPs

**TABLE 6-4. CONTRAINDICATIONS TO IUD USE**

| Absolute | Relative |
|---|---|
| Pregnancy | Prior ectopic pregnancy |
| Acute salpingitis/cervicitis | Dysmenorrhea |
| Dysfunctional uterine bleeding | |
| GU tract malignancy | |
| Anomalous intrauterine cavity | |
|   (e.g., multiple fibroids) | |

{ morbidity For IUD Use is  >  For OCP
{ Mortality For IUD Use is  <  For OCP

(5/1000 women-years and 1/1000 women-years, respectively), but the mortality is lower for IUD users (at 3 to 5 deaths/1,000,000 women-years).

## Insertion

Intrauterine devices are best inserted on the third or fourth day of an otherwise normal period to ensure that the patient is not pregnant at the time of insertion and because the dilated cervical os facilitates insertion. Should pregnancy occur while a patient is using an IUD, and pregnancy is to continue, the IUD should be removed if the string or lower portion of the device is visible.

This method of birth control requires little patient motivation at the potential expense of menstrual morbidity. The overall failure rate is about 2 to 4/100 women-years with the majority occurring during the first 30 days of use.

## SUMMARY OF REVERSIBLE CONTRACEPTIVE METHODS

See table 6.5 on page 216.

## STERILIZATION

Surgical sterilization as a method of contraception should be considered as irreversible. Reversible contraceptive methods tend to be used as a way of predictably spacing childbirth, whereas sterilization is more commonly selected by men and women who have attained their reproductive goals. A much smaller fraction of sterilization procedures are performed because of serious maternal illness making pregnancy extraordinarily hazardous and potentially fatal.

There are many methods of female sterilization ranging from hysterectomy to tubal ligation (laparotomy, minilaparotomy, laparoscopic electrocoagulation, and laparoscopic tubal plication, Tables 6-6 and 6-7). Hysterectomy as a sterilization procedure is only warranted when other indications exist for removal of the uterus, (e.g., pelvic or uterine disease).

**TABLE 6-5. SUMMARY OF REVERSIBLE CONTRACEPTIVE METHODS**

| Method | Partner Responsible | Failure Rate[a] (per 100 women-years) | Advantages | Disadvantages |
|---|---|---|---|---|
| OCP | Female | 0.3 | Lowest failure rate method | Side effects (see text) |
| IUD[b] | Female | 2–4 | Reliable; requires little attention | Menorrhagia; risk of salpingitis; pain |
| Periodic continence and BBT[c] | Both | 6.6 | No medication; no appliances required during coitus | Requires intelligence and cooperation |
| Diaphragm and jelly | Female | 12 | No systemic side effects | Requires constant motivation |
| Condom | Male | 13 | Protects against STD | Decreased sensation |
| Coitus interruptus | Male | 16 | Uncomplicated and inexpensive | Requires good ejaculatory control/high motivation |
| Vaginal foam | Female | 38 | Inexpensive and easy | High method failure rate; best used in combination |

"Morning-after" pills and induced abortion are by definition not forms of contraception. They act after conception and as such are forms of induced abortion. For further notes on induced abortion and sterilization see the appropriate section in the notes.

[a]The overall failure rate is a combination of both method failure (dependent on the relative simplicity of the technique), and patient failure (dependent primarily on patient motivation).

[b]The mechanism of action of IUDs is still uncertain. They may act after conception thus representing a form of induced abortion rather than contraception.

[c]Simple periodic continence (rhythm method) is based on unsubstantiated assumptions regarding timing of ovulation and sperm survival times. This is borne out by a high failure rate of 24/100 women-years.

**STD**, sexually transmitted disease.

**TABLE 6-6. SURGICAL STERILIZATION**

Methods of gaining peritoneal access for tubal sterilization
1. Laparoscope and trocar (for manipulator)
2. Posterior colpotomy (poor visualization)
3. "Minilaparotomy" (3 cm suprapubic incision)
4. Formal laparotomy (rarely required)
5. Hysteroscopy (experimental, obliterate fallopian tube ostia from within uterine cavity)

Currently laparoscopic tubal ligation using mechanical rings or clamps are most favored because they are least invasive and can be performed on an outpatient basis. Morbidity (~1.0% due to anesthesia, inadvertent cautery of abdominopelvic organs, pulmonary embolism) and mortality (4 to 8 per 100,000 procedures, most often attributable to anesthetic complications) rates for laparoscopic procedures are acceptably low.

Tubal ligation has a failure rate between 0.1 and 2.0% due to (1) patient failure-conception before the procedure, (2) method failure, poor surgical technique and recanalization.

Although there have been substantial advances in tubal reconstructive surgery (salpingoplasty), it is costly and results are uncertain. For this reason sterilization should not be performed on patients that are likely to want to become pregnant at a later date. Salpingoplasty also increases the risk of subsequent tubal pregnancy.

A posttubal ligation syndrome had been suggested consisting variably of menorrhagia, dysmenorrhea, and alterations in blood sex hormone levels. It has been demonstrated that in fact menstrual periods tend to be lighter after tubal sterilization; increased dysmenorrhea may complicate unipolar electrocautery; interruption of the utero-ovarian artery (within mesosalpinx) may be implicated in the change in serum sex hormone levels (usually subclinical).

Male sterilization by interruption of the vas deferens is technically simpler and associated with less morbidity and mortality than most forms of female sterilization (Table 6-8). Efficacy is equally high, however, adjunctive forms of contraception should be advised until two successive sperm samples are found to be devoid of sperm (weeks to months) while the

**TABLE 6-7. TUBAL STERILIZATION PROCEDURES**[a]

| Name | Description | Comment |
| --- | --- | --- |
| Irving | Divide tube[b]; free cut ends from mesosalpinx; bury proximal end in myometrium, lateral end in mesosalpinx | Lowest method failure rate |
| Pomeroy | Reabsorbable ligature placed around a knuckle of tube; divide tube | Simplest method with acceptable failure rate |
| Parkland | Separate 2.5 cm of tube from mesosalpinx (in an avascular plane); reabsorbable ligatures at either end of freed portion of tube; resect freed segment of tube | Method failure rate 1/400 |
| Kroener (fimbriectomy) | Doubly ligate ampullary end of tube proximal to resected fimbria | Method failure rate may be unacceptable (controversial) |
| Madlener | Crush base of a knuckle of tube; nonreabsorbable ligature applied | High (7%) method failure rate |

[a]Fallopian tubes are identified by visualization of fimbriated end while suspended from Babcock clamp; if tube is dropped during procedure, identification must be repeated.
[b]tube refers to fallopian tube.

distal vas deferens is emptied. The previously reported risk of autoimmune disease after vasectomy has not been substantiated, however, there still exists controversy over whether atherosclerosis may be accelerated in these patients.

# INDUCED ABORTION

Induced abortion is defined as a voluntary termination of pregnancy by any means before 20 weeks last menstrual period (LMP). The Canadian Medical Association (CMA) revised its policy regarding induced abortion in 1966. In

**TABLE 6-8. VASECTOMY**

| Description | Comment |
| --- | --- |
| Incise scrotum and spermatic fascia; resect 1–2 cm of vas deferens; ligate free ends of vas | Outpatient procedure; sterility not immediate (wks–mos delay) |

1970 sections 251 and 252 of the Criminal Code of Canada were modified based on the policies adopted by the CMA in 1967:

**CMA Policy (1967)**          **Modified Criminal Code (1970)**
Indications for induced abortion:

1. When continuation of the pregnancy may threaten the life or health of the mother
2. When there is a high likelihood of serious congenital malformation or illness
3. When pregnancy is the result of sexual assault

1. Accepted

2. Not accepted

3. Not accepted

In 1971 the CMA revised its position again to:

1. Include social grounds as an indication for induced abortion.
2. Eliminate "therapeutic abortion committees."
3. Request a legal definition for maternal "health."

In 1981 the CMA reviewed its position but made no further alterations in its policy. The Criminal Code has not been modified since 1970. The current CMA policy also,

**Supports**
1. The provision of at least one hospital per geographic region where induced abortions are made equally available to all women

**Opposes**
1. "Abortion-on-demand"
2. Abortion as a form of birth control

2. That no health care worker be compelled to participate in the procedure if it is contrary to their beliefs or wishes
3. That physicians inform patients if their moral/religious views restrict them from recommending induced abortion

In recognition that the optimal solution to the abortion dilemma is prevention of unwanted pregnancy the CMA suggests public education regarding birth control and responsible sexual behavior. In 1982 the induced abortion rate (excluding private clinics, illegal abortions, and those performed on Canadians in the United States) was 17.8 per 100 live births (~1 per 6 live births).

In 1973 the United States Supreme Court ruling in the Roe v. Wade case redefined what constitutes a legally acceptable abortion in the United States. The essence of the liberalization was that induced abortion was to be considered permissible if pregnancy threatened not only the life of the mother but also her health.

The indications for induced abortion currently propounded by the American College of Obstetricians are:

1. When continuation of the pregnancy may threaten the life of the mother or seriously impair her health;
2. When the pregnancy has resulted from rape or incest;
3. When continuation of the pregnancy is likely to result in the birth of a child with severe physical deformities or mental retardation.

In addition to the relatively minimal maternal mortality (0.6 per 100,000 induced abortions) the following effects on subsequent childbearing may be observed: (1) increased incidence of spontaneous midtrimester abortion, (2) increased incidence of preterm labor, (3) greater frequency of low birthweight infants (< 2.5 kg), and (4) infertility due to overzealous curettage (Asherman's syndrome). There are conflicting opinions as to whether the incidence of each of these complications is in fact higher after induced abortion. There is, however, almost universal agreement that any method of induced abortion that necessitates vigorous cervical dilatation is more frequently attended by subsequent cervical incompetence.

## Techniques for Induced Abortion

### Surgical (4–14 wk LMP)
Cervical dilatation and (1) curettage or
                    (2) vacuum aspiration
(with or without prior laminaria tent for enhanced cervical dilatation).
Laparotomy for (1) hysterotomy or
                (2) hysterectomy.

### Medical (> 16 wk LMP)
Intra-amnionic hyperosmolar fluids: (1) 20% saline or
                                 (2) 30% urea.
Prostaglandin $F_{2\alpha}$ or prostaglandin analogues by
(1) Intra-amnionic injection,
(2) Extraovular injection,
(3) Vaginal suppositories,
(4) Parenteral injection,
(5) Oral ingestion.
Various combinations of the above methods are also used.

# 7

# Human Sexuality

A brief description of the four phases of the physiologic sexual response cycle (as described by Masters and Johnson) and brief mention of the more common forms of sexual dysfunction are provided here. For a more detailed overview of this topic the reader may consult Dickes and Simons: *Understanding Human Behavior in Health and Illness* (Tables 7-1 and 7-2).

Sexual dysfunction is much more common and less ominous than previously thought, that is the presence of sexual dysfunction does not always imply serious underlying psychopathology. The two most common forms of female sexual dysfunction are general sexual dysfunction (frigidity, the inability to experience erotic pleasure upon stimulation) and orgastic dysfunction (the inability to attain orgasm through sexual intercourse). The two most frequent forms of male sexual dysfunction include premature ejaculation (the lack of voluntary control over the ejaculatory reflex once sexually aroused) and erectile dysfunction (inability to attain or sustain an erect penis upon stimulation).

One must always rule out organic disorders (e.g., Leriche syndrome, diabetic neuropathy) and drug adverse reactions as the cause of sexual dysfunction. Drugs most prone to cause sexual dysfunction are agents that interfere with the function of the autonomic nervous system (e.g., many antihypertensives) and heterosexual sex steroids that are occasionally administered therapeutically for other illnesses.

At least as important as this factual knowledge is the ability to obtain an adequate history, which requires a mature, nonjudgmental interviewer capable of dealing with patients on their own level in a candid, honest manner.

**TABLE 7-1. MALE SEXUAL RESPONSE CYCLE**

| Excitement (min–hr) | Plateau (30 sec–3 min) | Orgasmic (3–15 sec) | Resolution (10–15 min) |
| --- | --- | --- | --- |
| **Skin** | | | |
| No change | Inconstant morbilliform erythema, "sexual flush" | No change | Disappears |
| **Penis** | | | |
| Erection within 10–30 sec | Deepened coloration of glans; shaft and glans enlarge | 3–4 major contractions @ 0.8 sec intervals followed by minor contractions | Partial involution within 5–10 sec; complete detumescence within 30 min; variable duration refractoriness |
| **Scrotum/Testes** | | | |
| Scrotum tightens; testes ascends | Testicular enlargement due to vascular congestion | No change | Return to normal within 30 min |
| **Other** | | | |
| Inconstant nipple erection | Mucoid preejaculate containing viable sperm secreted; heart rate, BP and respirations increase | Partial loss of voluntary muscular control; further increase in vital signs | Return to normal within 10 min |

Physicians must refrain from permitting their personal views from interfering with the professional services they have been engaged to render.

All physicians should be aware of the reputable resources available within their communities for the therapy of sexual dysfunction.

Finally, when faced with an immature, seductive or otherwise sexually aggressive patient, physicians should be able to recognize the situation and deal with it appropriately.

**TABLE 7-2. FEMALE SEXUAL RESPONSE CYCLE**

| Excitement (min–hr) | Plateau (30 sec–3 min) | Orgasmic (3–15 sec) | Resolution (10–15 min) |
|---|---|---|---|
| **Skin** | | | |
| No change | Inconstant morbilliform erythema "sexual flush" | No change | Disappears |
| **Breasts** | | | |
| Nipple erection; venous congestion; areolar enlargement | Progression of congestion and areolar enlargement | No change | Return to normal |
| **Clitoris** | | | |
| Glans and shaft diameter increase | Shaft retracts within swollen prepuce | No change | Normal position resumed within 10 sec; full detumescence within 10 min |
| **Labia Majora** | | | |
| Nullip Flatten | May swell if this phase unduly prolonged | No change | Resume normal size within 2 min |
| Multip Rapid congestion | Further enlargement | No change | Resume normal size within 15 min |
| **Labia Minora** | | | |
| Increase size 2–3x normal | Further enlargement | Proximal contractions in synchrony with lower one third vagina | Return to normal within 5 min |
| Nullip Pink | Red | | |
| Multip Red | Dark red | | |
| **Vagina** | | | |
| Copious transudative lubricant fluid | Transudate continues to form throughout this phase | No change | Pools on vaginal floor of upper two thirds (supine position) |

**TABLE 7-2.** (*Continued*)

| Excitement (min–hr) | Plateau (30 sec–3 min) | Orgasmic (3–15 sec) | Resolution (10–15 min) |
|---|---|---|---|
| **Vagina upper two thirds** | | | |
| Dilates; rugae flatten; and vaginal wall lengthens as uterus rises | Further dilatation | No change | Cervix descends into seminal pool within 3–4 min (supine pos) |
| **Vagina lower one third** | | | |
| Lumen dilates; walls become congested | Contraction around penis aids in thrusting action on clitoral shaft via labia and prepuce | 3–15 contractions @3/4 sec intervals | Congestion disappears in seconds |
| **Uterus** | | | |
| Ascends into false pelvis | Strong sustained contractions | Contractions persist | Slow return to normal |
| **Rectum** | | | |
| | | Inconstant rhythmic contractions | Cease within seconds |

*Multip*, multipara; *Nullip*, nullipara.

# Bibliography

Oxorn H: Human Labor and Birth, 4th ed. New York, N.Y.: Appleton-Century-Crofts, 1980

Danforth DN: Obstetrics and Gynecology, 3rd ed. Hagerstown, Md.: Harper & Row, 1977

Pritchard JA: Williams Obstetrics, 17th ed. East Norwalk, Conn.: Appleton-Century-Crofts, 1985

Jones HW: Novak's Textbook of Gynecology, 10th ed. Baltimore, Md.: Williams and Wilkins, 1981

Moore KL: The Developing Human, 2nd ed. Philadelphia, Pa.: WB Saunders, 1977

Speroff L: Clinical Gynecologic Endocrinology and Infertility, 2nd ed. Baltimore, Md.: Williams and Wilkins, 1978

Smith DR: General Urology, 10th ed. Los Altos, Ca.: Lange Medical Publications, 1981

Wolfman W, Holtz G: Update on ectopic pregnancy. CMAJ 129:1265, 1983

Oral contraceptive pill review: Medical Letter 26:67, 1984

Sexually transmitted diseases, treatment: Medical Letter 28:23, 1986

Hughes JG: Synopsis of Pediatrics, 5th ed. St. Louis, Mo.: CV Mosby, 1980

Gosink BB: Exercises in Diagnostic Radiology, 2nd ed. (#8 Diagnostic Ultrasound). Philadelphia, Pa.: WB Saunders, 1981

Caplan R: Principle of Obstetrics. Baltimore, Md.: Williams and Wilkins, pp 265–80, 1982

Freinkel N, Dooley S, Metzger B: Care of the pregnant woman with insulin-dependent diabetes mellitus. N Engl J Med 313:96, 1985

Sullivan J, Ramanathan K: Management of medical problems in pregnancy—Severe cardiac disease. N Engl J Med 313:304, 1985

Mushlin A: Diagnostic tests in breast cancer. Ann Int Med 103:79, 1985

Health and Public Policy Committee, American College of Physicians: The use of diagnostic tests for screening and evaluating breast lesions. Ann Intern Med 103:143, 1985

Keen H, Ng Tang Fui S: The definition and classification of diabetes mellitus. Clin Endo Met 11:279, 1982

Perloff J: Pregnancy and cardiovascular disease in heart disease, a Textbook of Cardiovascular Medicine, 2nd ed. Philadelphia, Pa.: WB Saunders, pp. 1763–81, 1984

Dickes R, Simons RC: Adult sexuality. In Understanding Human Behavior in Health and Illness. Baltimore, Md.: Williams and Wilkins, 213–82, 1977

Woods D: Oral contraceptives, 1985: A synopsis. CMAJ 133:463, 1985

CMA Policy Summary: Abortion. CMAJ 133:318A, 1985

Lindheimer M, Katz A: Hypertension in pregnancy. N Engl J Med 313:675, 1985

Rizack M, Hillman C: The Medical Letter Handbook of Drug Interactions. New Rochelle, N.Y.: The Medical Letter, pp 42–5, 1983

# Index

A/B/O blood group incompatibility, 64–65
Abdominal examination
  cephalopelvic disproportion and, 87
  neonatal, 38
Abortion
  cytogenetic studies and, 77
  induced, 219–221
  prenatal history and, 26
  vaginal bleeding and, 44
Abortus, 105
Abruptio placentae, 45
  management of, 47–48
Abscess, salpingitis and, 126
Acanthoadenocarcinoma, 167
Adenitis, 111
Adenoacanthoma, 158
Adenocarcinoma, cervical, 143
Adenohypophyseal necrosis, 48
Adenomatous endometrial hyperplasia, 155–156
Adenomyosis, 132–133
Adenosis, vaginal, 122
Adnexal torsion, 128
Adrenal cortex, 18
Adrenal enzyme deficiency, 9–10

Adrenal rest tumor, 176
Adrenarche, 179
Adrenergic agonist, beta, 92
Afterpains, 40
Agenesis, gonadal, 7
Airway in neonatal resuscitation, 34–35
Albuminoid crystals, Reinke's, 171
Allantois, 3
Alpha-fetoprotein, 174
Amenorrhea, 184–191
  oral contraceptives and, 207
Amniocentesis, 76–77
Amniotic fluid
  amniocentesis and, 76–77
  bilirubin and, 77
  embolism and, 52
Amniotic membrane rupture
  labor and, 32
  premature, 95–97
Amniotomy, 32
Androgens, 134
Anemia, 27–28
Aneuploidy, 77
Anosmia, 191
Anovulation, 197–199

Antacids, 28
Anti Rh$^+$ antibody, 63
Anticoagulation, maternal, 74
Antisperm antibodies, 193, 194
Aortic stenosis, 72
Apgar score, 36, 37
Apocrine sweat gland adenitis, 111
Appearance in neonatal assessment,
    38
Appendicitis, 127
ARM. *See* Artificial rupture of amnio-
    tic membranes
Arrhenoblastoma cell tumor, 171–172
Arrhythmia, 73–74
Artificial rupture of amniotic mem-
    branes (ARM), 32
ASA, 92
Asherman's syndrome, 188
Asphyxia, neonatal, 36
Aspiration, breast and, 141
Assessment
    fetal well-being, 75–89
    neonatal, 35–38
Atenolol, 58
Atony, uterine, 50
Atrophic striae, 20
Attitude, 88
Autosomal recessive disorder, 9

Bacterial endocarditis, 71, 73
Bacteriuria, 75
Ballottement, 23
Bartholin duct neoplasia, 118
Bartholinitis, 111
Basal body temperature (BBT), 199
BBT. *See* Basal body temperature
Beat-to-beat variability, 80–81

Behçet's syndrome, 107, 109
Benign cystic teratoma, 175
Beta adrenergic agonist, 92
Beta-human chorionic gonadotropin
    embryonal carcinoma and, 174
    trophoblastic disease and, 103–104
Bilirubin, 77
Biopsy
    cone, 145
    testicular, 193
Birth
    mortality and, 105
    preterm, 26
    term, 25
Birth control, 205–221
    abortion and, 218–221
    intrauterine device and, 213–215
    oral contraceptives and, 205–213
Bladder, 21
Bleeding
    chorioadenoma destruens and, 101
    choriocarcinoma and, 102
    dysfunctional uterine, 195–204
    fetal, 48
    ovulation, 128
    pregnancy and, 38–48
    vaginal
        postmenopausal, 159
        pregnancy and, 43–53, 201–202
Bleeding diathesis
    dysfunctional uterine bleeding and,
        199
    postpartum hemorrhage and, 51
Blighted ovum, 44
Blindness, 57
Blood. *See also* Bleeding
    fetal scalp, 76
    pregnancy and, 16

Blood flow, renal, 56
Blood group incompatibility
   A/B/O, 64–65
   Rh, 61–64
Blood pressure
   normal pregnancy and, 15
   pregnancy-induced hypertension
      and, 53–60
Blood test, 26
Bloody tap, amniocentesis and, 76–77
Body
   Call-Exner, 170–178
   Donovan, 114
   psammoma, 164
Body weight, 198
Bone resorption, 183
Borderline mucinous cystadenocar-
      cinoma, 166
Borderline papillary cystadenocar-
      cinoma, 165
Bowen's disease, 113
Braxton-Hicks contractions, 24
Breast
   carcinoma and, 139–141
   distension of, 28–29
   lesion detection and evaluation, 142
   postpartum period and, 39
   pregnancy and, 20
Brenner tumor, 163–164, 167


CABG. *See* Coronary arterial bypass
      grafting
Calcification of fibroid, 151
Calcium gluconate, 60
Call-Exner bodies, 170–178
*Calymmatobacterium granulomatis*,
   114

Canadian Medical Association policy
   on abortion, 218–220
Canal, Nuck's, 118
Cancer. *See* Malignancy
*Candida*
   vaginitis and, 120
   vulva and, 108
Carbohydrate metabolism, 209–210
Carcinoid tumor, ovarian, 175
Carcinoma
   breast, 139–141
   cervical, 141–147
   choriocarcinoma, 101–105
   embryonal, 173–174
   endometrial, 157–160
   vaginal, 123
Carcinoma-in-situ
   cervix and, 143
   vaginal, 123
   vulva and, 113
Cardiac disease in pregnancy, 69–74
Cardiomyopathy, 72
Cardiovascular system
   neonatal assessment and, 38
   normal pregnancy and, 14
Carnerous fibroid, 151
Catheterization, cardiac, 70
Cephalopelvic disproportion (CPD),
      87–88, 89
Cerclage, cervical, 94–95
Cervix
   antisperm antibodies and, 193,
      194
   bleeding in pregnancy and, 44
   carcinoma and, 141–147
   colposcopy and, 147–149
   dilation of, during labor, 31
   incompetent, 94–95

Cervix (*cont.*)
  intraepithelial neoplasia and, 143,
    145
  mucus and
    infertility and, 193
    ovulation and, 196
  myoma and, 150
  polyps and, 200
  postpartum period and, 39
  pregnancy and, 22
  ripening of, 31
Chadwick's sign, 20
Chancroid, 114
Chlamydial disease, 114
  salpingitis and, 125
  urethral, 113
Chorioadenoma destruens, 101
Choriocarcinoma, 101–105
  ovary and, 174
Chorionic gonadotropin, human, 23
  embryonal carcinoma and, 174
  pregnancy and, 136
  trophoblastic disease and, 103–104
Chromosomal aberration, 77
Chromosomal sex, 3
Cicatrization of fallopian tube, 192–
    193
Circulatory disease, vulvar, 109
Clear cell tumor, 167
Cloaca, 3
Clonidine, 183
Coagulation, disseminated
    intravascular
  fetal death and, 25
  postpartum hemorrhage and, 51–
    52
Coelomic epithelium, 4
  ovarian neoplasm and, 163
Coincident hypertension, 54–55

Colloid, 58–59
Colostrum, 39
Colposcopy, 147–149
  cervical carcinoma and, 145
Colpotomy, 127
Condyloma accuminatum, 112
Cone biopsy, 145
Contraception, 204–221
  abortion as, 218–221
  intrauterine device and, 213–215
  oral, 205–213
    anovulatory cycle and, 197
Contraction stress test, 79–82
Contractions, Braxton-Hicks, 24
Convulsions
  eclaptic, 59–60
  pregnancy-induced hypertension
    and, 56
Cord, umbilical, 33
Coronary arterial bypass grafting
    (CABG), 73
Corporeal myoma, 150
Corpus luteum
  cyst and, 169
  pregnancy and, 18
Corrected heart disease, 73–74
Cortex, adrenal, 18
Cortical sex cords, 4
CPD. *See* Cephalopelvic disproportion
Crowning, 33
Cryptorchidism, 7
Crystals, Reinke's albuminoid, 171
Culdocentesis, 136
Cyanotic heart disease, 72
Cycle
  menstrual, 154
  sexual response, 224–226
Cystadenocarcinoma
  borderline mucinous, 166

endometrioid, 167
  malignant, 166
Cystadenofibroma, ovarian, 164–165
Cystadenoma
  endometrioid, 167
  mucinous, 165–166
Cystic endometrial hyperplasia, 155–156
Cystic fibroid, 151
Cystic ovary, 168–170
Cystic teratoma, 175
Cystic vulvar neoplasia, 118
Cystocoele, 138
Cytogenetic studies, 77


Dactinomycin, 104
Danazol, 134
Death. *See* Mortality
Defemininization, 172
Degeneration, hydropic, 101
Dehydrotestosterone (DHT), 7
Delivery
  normal, 33–35
  preterm, 91, 92–93
  Rh incompatibility and, 63–64
Denominator, 88
Dermatitis, vulva, 108
Dermoid cyst, 175
Descent, delivery and, 33
DHT. *See* Dehydrotestosterone
Diabetes mellitus (DM)
  gestational, 67
  maternal, 65–69
Diathesis
  dysfunctional uterine bleeding and, 199
  postpartum hemorrhage and, 51

Diazoxide, 58
Digital vaginal examination, 27
Dilation, cervical, 31
Discoloration, vaginal, 20
Disseminated intravascular coagulation
  fetal death and, 25
  postpartum hemorrhage and, 51–52
Diuresis, postpartum period and, 40
Diuretic, thiazide, 57
Diverticulum, metanephric, 1
Dizygotic twins, 98
DM. *See* Diabetes
Donovan bodies, 114
Drug interactions with oral contraceptives, 211
DUB. *See* Dysfunctional uterine bleeding
Duct
  Bartholin, 118
  gonadal, 7
  mesonephric, 1–2
  wolffian, 3
Dysfunctional uterine bleeding (DUB), 195–202
  infertility and, 192
Dysgenesis
  müllerian, 188
  ovarian, 188–189
Dysgerminoma, 172–173
Dysmenorrhea, 202–203
  secondary, 123–136
Dyspareunia, 123
  menopause and, 183
Dysphoria, 42
Dysplasia
  cervical, 144
  colposcopy and, 147–148
Dystocia, 84–89
Dystrophy, vulvar, 109

Early decelerations, 81
Ecbolic maneuvers, 32
Eclampsia, 53, 59–60
Ectopic pregnancy, 134–136
    pain and, 128
Ectopy
    gonadal, 7
    renal, 2
Edema, 53, 56
Edematous chorionic villi, grapelike, 102
Eisenmenger's syndrome, 73
Ejaculation dysfunction, 194
Electrocardiography, fetal heart rate and, 80–81
Embolism
    amniotic fluid, 52
    pulmonary trophoblastic, 103
Embryology, genitourinary, 1–12. See also Genitourinary embryology
Embryonal carcinoma, 173–174
Embryonic rests, 176
Emesis, 21
Emphysematous vaginitis, 120
End diastolic pressure, 14
Endocarditis, 71, 73
Endocrine system. See Hormone
Endoderm, 4
Endometrioid cystadenoma, 167
Endometriosis, 132–134
    pain and, 128
    vagina and, 122
    vulva and, 118
Endometritis
    amenorrhea and, 187–188
    dysfunctional uterine bleeding and, 200

salpingitis and, 125
Endometrium
    carcinoma and, 157–160
    hyperplasia and, 153–157
    oral contraceptives and, 206
    polyps and, 157
    dysfunctional uterine bleeding and, 200
Engagement, 31
Enzyme deficiency, adrenal, 9–10
Epithelial cell analysis, 78
Epithelium, coelomic, 4
    ovarian neoplasm and, 163
Erythrocyte sedimentation rate (ESR), 40
Erythromycin, 113
Erythroplasia of Queyrat, 113
ESR. See Erythrocyte sedimentation rate
Estriols, 75–76
Estrogen
    amenorrhea and, 184, 186
    anovulatory cycle and, 197
    menopause and, 182–183
    obesity and, 155
    oral contraceptives and, 205–206, 207, 209
    pregnancy and, 14
    vaginal adenosis and, 122
Evaluation. See Assessment
Exchange transfusion, 62–63
Exhaustion, maternal, 89
Extension, delivery and, 33
External genitalia, 7–12
External rotation, delivery and, 34
Extracellular fluid, 55–56
Extraembryonal teratomatous germ cell tumor, 174–176

Extremities, neonatal assessment of, 38

Fallopian tube
infertility and, 192–193
inflammation of, 124–132
False labor, 91
Fascia, paracervical, 138
Fatty fibroid, 151
Female pseudohermaphroditism, 9
Female sexual response scycle, 225–226
Ferning of cervical mucus, 196
Fertility, 191–194
Fetal heart rate, 79–82
Fetopelvic relations, 88
Fetopelvic ultrasound, 78
α-Fetoprotein, 174
Fetus
blood loss and, 48
death of, 25, 105
exchange transfusion and, 62, 64
gestational age of, 83
hemolytic disease and, 60–65
maternal anticoagulation and, 74
maturity indices and, 78–82
pregnancy-induced hypertension and, 57–58
respiratory distress syndrome and, 93–94
sulphonamide and, 74
tetracycline and, 74
well-being of, 75–89
Fibroadenoma, ovarian, 164
Fibroid, 149–153
Fibroma, 171
Fine-needle aspiration of breast, 141

Fistula, rectourethral, 3
Fitz-Hugh-Curtis syndrome, 126
Flexion, delivery and, 33
Fluid
amniotic
amniocentesis and, 76–77
bilirubin and, 77
embolism and, 52
extracellular, 55–56
retention of, 14
Folate, 27–28
Follicle cyst, 168–169
Follicle-stimulating hormone (FSH)
amenorrhea and, 187
menopause and, 181–182
pregnancy and, 23
Forewaters, 32
Fox-Fordyce disease, 111
Friedman curves, 85, 86
Fundus, uterine, 41

Gamete, 192
Gardnerella vaginalis, 120
Gartner's duct cyst, 118, 122
Gastrointestinal system
oral contraceptives and, 210–211
pregnancy and, 15–16
GDM. See Gestational diabetes mellitus
Genitalia, 7–12
Genitourinary system
embryology and, 1–12
external genitalia and, 7–12
gonadal unit and, 3–7, 7
nephritic unit and, 1–2
vesicourethral unit and, 3
neonatal assessment of, 38

Genitourinary system (*cont.*)
pregnancy and, 15–16
vaginal bleeding and, 43
Germ cell tumor
primordial, 172–176
teratomatous, 174–176
Gestational age, 90
ultrasound and, 83
Gestational diabetes mellitus (GDM), 67
Gestational trophoblastic disease (GTD), 100–105
Gingivitis, 21
Gland. *See also* Hormone
pituitary, 16–17
vulvar, 111
Glomerular filtration rate, 67–68
Glucocorticoid
pregnancy and, 20
respiratory distress syndrome and, 94
Glucose
diabetes and, 65
oral contraceptive and, 209–210
Glucose tolerance test, 66
Glycosuria, 40
Goddell's sign, 22
Gonadal insufficiency, 187
Gonadal mesenchyme, 168
Gonadal unit, 3–7
Gonadotropin, human chorionic, 23
embryonal carcinoma and, 174
pregnancy and, 136
trophoblastic disease and, 103–104
Gonococcal disease, 113
salpingitis and, 124
Granuloma inguinale, 114
Granulosa cell tumor, 170–171

Grapelike edematous chorionic villi, 102
Gravidity, 25
Growth retardation, intrauterine, 84
GTD. *See* Gestational trophoblastic disease
Gubernaculum, 5–6
Gynandroblastoma, 172

HAI urine test, 23
HCG. *See* Human chorionic gonadotropin
Head, neonatal, 38
Headache, 57
Heart
neonatal assessment of, 38
normal pregnancy and, 14
Heart disease, 69–74
Heart rate, fetal, 79–82
Hegar's sign, 22
Hemolytic disease of newborn, 60–65
*Hemophilus ducreyi*, 114
Hemorrhage. *See* Bleeding
Heparin, 74
Hepatobiliary system, 210
Hermaphroditism, 9–12
Herpes genitalis, 112
Herpes simplex virus, 120
Heterosexual precocious puberty, 180
Heyman packing, 160
High-risk pregnancy, 27
Hilus cell tumor, 171
Hormone
amenorrhea and, 184–187
dysfunctional uterine bleeding and, 198
endometrial hyperplasia and, 155

endometriosis and, 133–134
infertility and, 194
labor and, 30
menopause and, 181
pregnancy and, 16–17
puberty and, 179–180
Human chorionic gonadotropin
    (HCG), 23
embryonal carcinoma and, 174
pregnancy and, 136
trophoblastic disease and, 103–104
Human milk, 39
Hyaline fibroid, 151
Hydatidiform mole, 101
    ultrasound and, 84
Hydradenitis, 111
Hydralazine, 58
Hydrocele, 118
Hydropic degeneration, 101
Hydrops fetalis, 61–62
21-Hydroxylase deficiency, 9
Hymen, 3
Hypermenorrhea, 152
Hyperpigmentation, 20
Hyperplasia
    endometrial, 153–157, 159
    vulvar, 110
Hyperprolactinemia, 186
Hyperreflexia, 57
Hyperstimulation, 81–82
Hypertension
    pregnancy-induced, 26, 53–60
    pulmonary, 73
Hypertonic uterine insufficiency, 87
Hypertrophic cardiomyopathy, 72
Hypogenesis, gonadal, 7
Hypomenorrhea, 195
Hypothyroidism, 187

Hypotonic uterine insufficiency, 85
Hysterectomy, 145–146

Immunization, rubella, 42
Immunoglobulin, Rh, 42
In utero fetal exchange transfusion,
    62, 64
Inclusion cyst, vaginal, 122
Incompetent cervix, 94–95
Indifferent gonad, 4
Indomethacin, 92, 93
Induced abortion
    as birth control, 219–221
    cytogenetic studies and, 77
Infection
    amenorrhea and, 187–188
    fallopian tube and, 124–132
    fibroid and, 151
    postpartum hemorrhage and, 52–53
    vaginitis, 21, 118–122
Infertility, 191–194
Inflammation
    fallopian tube and, 124–132
    pyelonephritis and, 74
    vulvar, 107
Intermenstrual bleeding, 195
Internal rotation, delivery and, 33
Intraepithelial neoplasia, cervical,
    143, 145
Intrauterine device (IUD), 127
Intrauterine growth retardation
    (IUGR), 84
Intravascular coagulation,
    disseminated
    fetal death and, 25
    postpartum hemorrhage and, 51–
    52

Intravascular extracellular fluid
(IVECF), 55–56
Intravenous leiomyomatosis, 150
Iron deficiency anemia, 27
Ischemic heart disease, 73–74
Isoimmunization, 60
Isosexual precocious puberty, 180
Isoxuprine, 92, 93
IUD. *See* Intrauterine device
IUGR. *See* Intrauterine growth
retardation
IVECF. *See* Intravascular extracellular
fluid

Jaundice, 60–65

Karyotyping, 77
Keratitis, 108
Kernicterus, 62
Ketonuria, 40
Kidney
embryology and, 1–2
pregnancy-induced hypertension
and, 56
pyelonephritis and, 74
Kraurosis, 109

L/S ratio. *See* Lecithin/sphingomyelin
ratio
Labor
dystocia and, 84–89
normal, 30–35
preterm, 90–97
Laceration, 50
Lactation, 39–40

Lactoferrin, 39
Laparoscopy
ectopic pregnancy and, 136
salpingitis and, 127
Large for gestational age (LGA), 90
Last menstrual period (LMP)
diagnosis of pregnancy and, 24
pregnancy and, 17, 22
Late decelerations, 81
Laxative, 28
Lecithin/sphingomyelin ratio (L/S
ratio), 78
respiratory distress syndrome and,
94
Leiomyoma, 149–153
Leopold's maneuvers, 26–27
Leukocytosis, 40
Leukoplakia, 117
Leydig cell tumor, 171
LFI urine test, 23
LGA. *See* Large for gestational age
Lichen sclerosis atrophicus (LSA),
109
Lie, 88
Ligament
round, 29
uterine prolapse and, 138
Ligation, tubal, 215, 217
Lightening, 31
Linea nigra, 20
Lipid cell tumor, 176
Lipid metabolism, 210
Live birth
mortality and, 105
prenatal history and, 26
Lochia, 40
Low birth weight infant, 90
LSA. *See* Lichen sclerosis atrophicus

Lung
  lecithin/sphingomyelin ratio and, 78
  respiratory distress syndrome and,
    93–94
Luteinizing hormone (LH)
  amenorrhea and, 184–185, 186–
    187
  menopause and, 181–182
  pregnancy and, 23
Luteoma, pregnancy, 170
Lymphogranuloma venereum, 114
Lysozyme, 39


Macrocytic anemia, 27–28
Magnesium sulfate, 59
Male pseudohermaphroditism, 11–12
Male sexual response cycle, 224
Malignancy
  breast and, 139–141
  carcinoma-in-situ and
    cervix and, 143
    vaginal, 123
    vulva and, 113
  choriocarcinoma and, 101–105
  embryonal, 173–174
  endometrial, 157–160
  ovarian, 160–178
  vaginal, 123
  vulva and, 113–115, 117
Malrotation, renal, 2
Mammography, 139–141
Maneuvers of Leopold, 26–27
Marginal sinus rupture, 46, 48
Mask of pregnancy, 20
Maternal estriols, 75–76
Maternal mortality rate, 106
Maturity indices, fetal, 78–82

Meconium, 32
Medullary sex cords, 4
Meigs' syndrome, 167
  ovarian neoplasm and, 176–177
  thecoma and, 171
Melasma, 20
Membranes, amniotic, 32, 95–97
Menarche, 179
Menometrorrhagia, 195
Menopause, 181–183
Menses
  amenorrhea and, 184–191
  cessation of, 181–183
  endometrium and, 154
  infection and, 125–126
  postpartum period and, 39
Mesenchyme
  gonadal, 4, 168
  metanephric, 1
Mesonephric tubule, 7
Mesonephroid type tumor, 167
Mesonephros, 1, 4
Metanephros, 1
Metastatic myoma, 150
Metastatic tumor, 177–178
Methotrexate, 104
Methyldopa, 58
Metoprolol, 58
Metorrhagia, 152
MIF. See Mullerian inhibiting factor
Milk, human, 39
Mitral stenosis, 72
Mixed epithelial ovarian tumor,
    164
Mole, hydatidiform, 101
  ultrasound and, 84
Molluscum contagiosum, 112
Molluscum fibrosum gravidarum, 21

Monozygotic pregnancy, 97–98
Montgomery's tubercles, 20
Mortality
    fetal, 83
    intrauterine device and, 214
    obstetric, 105–106
    oral contraceptive and, 212
Mucinous cyst, vulvar, 118
Mucinous cystadenocarcinoma, 166
Mucinous cystadenoma, 165–166
Mucosa, vaginal, 20
Mucus, cervical, 193
Müllerian duct, 7
Müllerian dysgenesis, 188
Müllerian inhibiting factor (MIF), 7
Multiple follicle cyst, 169
Multiple pregnancy, 97–100
    ultrasound and, 84
Muscle sheath, 138
Musculoskeletal system, 16
*Mycoplasma*, 125
Myoma, 149–153
    dysfunctional uterine bleeding and,
    200

Nausea, 21
Neck, 38
Necrosis
    adenohypophyseal, 48
    fibroid and, 151
*Neisseria gonorrhoeae*, 120
Neonate
    assessment of, 35–38
    hemolytic disease and, 60–65
    mortality and, 105–106
    polycystic kidney and, 2
    resuscitation of, 34–35, 37

Neoplasia. *See also* Malignancy
    cervical intraepithelial, 143, 145
    ovarian, 160–178
    pituitary, 189–190
    vulva and, 113–115, 117, 118–119
Nephritic unit, 1–2
Neurologic examination, 38
Neuropsychiatric effects, 210
Nipple secretion, 140
Nonsteroidal antiinflammatory drugs,
    203
Nonstress test of fetal well-being, 79–
    82
19-Norestosterones, 206
Nuck's canal, 118

Obesity, 155
Obstetrics. *See also* Pregnancy
    fetal well-being and, 75–89
    gestational trophoblastic disease
    and, 100–105
    hemolytic disease of newborn and,
    60–65
    mortality and, 105–106
    normal pregnancy and, 13–42
    prolapsed umbilical cord and, 89–
    90
Obstruction, fallopian tube, 192–193
OCP. *See* Oral contraceptive
OCT. *See* Oxytocin challenge test
Oligomenorrhea, 195
Oral contraceptive (OCP), 204–213
    anovulatory cycle and, 197
Oral glucose tolerance test, 66
Osteoporosis, 183
Ovary
    amenorrhea and, 186

dysgenesis and, 188–189
neoplasia and, 160–178
polycystic, 155
  dysfunctional uterine bleeding
    and, 198
  resistant, 187
  trophoblastic disease and, 102–103
Ovulation
  cervical mucus and, 196
  dysfunctional uterine bleeding and,
    199–201
  evidence of, 192
  hemorrhage and, 128
Ovum, blighted, 44
Oxytocin challenge test (OCT), 79–82


Packing
  Heyman, 160
  uterine, 50
Paget's disease, 113
Pain
  myoma and, 152
  pregnancy-induced hypertension
    and, 57
  round ligament syndrome and, 29
Palpation, 23
Papanicolaou smear, 145
Papillary cystadenocarcinoma, 165
Papillary cystadenoma, 164
Paracervical fascia, 138
Paramesonephric duct, 7
PCOD. *See* Polycystic ovarian disease
Pelvic kidney, 2
Pelvic pain, 123–136
  round ligament syndrome and, 29
Pelvic sonography, 83–84
Perinatal mortality, 105

Peritonitis, 126
Physiologic changes in pregnancy,
  13–16
Pigmentation, 20
PIH. *See* Pregnancy-induced
  hypertension
Piskacek's sign, 22
Pituitary gland
  neoplasm and, 189–190
  pregnancy and, 16–17
Placenta
  delivery of, 35
  normal pregnancy and, 17
  retained, 51
  traction of, 50
  ultrasound and, 83–84
Placenta previa, 45
  management of, 47
Plasma alpha-fetoprotein, 174
Plasma glucose, 65
PMT. *See* Premenstrual tension
  syndrome
Polycystic kidney, neonatal, 2
Polycystic ovarian disease (PCOD),
  155
Polycystic ovarian disease (POD)
  dysfunctional uterine bleeding and,
    198
Polyhydramnios, 84
Polymenorrhea, 195
Polyp
  cervical, 200
  endometrial, 157, 200
Polyzygotic pregnancy, 98
Position, delivery and, 88
Postcoital test, 194
Postmenopausal period
  bleeding and, 159, 195

Postmenopausal period (*cont.*)
  osteoporosis and, 183
  urethritis and, 113
  vaginitis and, 120
Postpartum period
  exchange transfusion and, 64
  hemorrhage and, 48–53
Postterm labor, 90
Precocious puberty, 180
Pregnancy
  cervical carcinoma and, 146–147
  diabetes and, 65–69
  dysfunctional uterine bleeding and,
    201–202
  ectopic, 134–136
    pain and, 128
  fetal well-being and, 75–89
  heart disease and, 69–74
  hemolytic disease of newborn and,
    60–65
  hypertension and, 53–60
  leiomyoma and, 152–153
  luteomas and, 170
  molar, 101
  mortality and, 105–106
  multiple pregnancy and, 97–100
  physiologic changes in, 13–16
  preterm labor and, 90–97
  prolapsed cord and, 89–90
  vaginal bleeding and, 43–53
Pregnancy-induced hypertension, 53–
  60
Premature rupture of membranes
  (PROM), 95–97
Premenstrual tension syndrome
  (PMT), 203–204
Prenatal care, 25–30
Prenatal virilization, 7

Presentation, 88
Presenting part, 88
Preterm delivery
  prenatal history and, 26
  Rh incompatibility and, 63–64
Preterm labor, 30, 90–97
Primary sex cord, 4
Primordial germ cell, 172–176
Primordial gonad, 5
Progestational effect of oral contracep-
  tives, 206
Progesterone
  dysfunctional uterine bleeding and,
    199
  normal pregnancy and, 16, 17
Progestins, 133–134
Prolactin, 185
Prolapse
  umbilical cord and, 89–90
  uterovaginal, 137–139
PROM. *See* Premature rupture of
  membranes
Pronephros, 1
Prophylaxis, endocarditis and, 71, 73
Propranolol, 58
Prostaglandin synthetase inhibitors, 92
Proteinuria
  hypertension and, 56
  pregnancy and, 53
Pruritus, vulvar, 117
Psammoma body, 164
Pseudohermaphroditism, 9–12
Pseudomyxoma peritoneii, 166
Psoriasis, vulvar, 108
Puberty, 179–181
  dysfunctional uterine bleeding and,
    197
  virilization and, 7, 9

Puerperal pain, 41
Puerperium, 38–42
Pulmonary embolus, trophoblastic, 103
Pulmonary hypertension, 73
Pulmonary vascular resistance, 73
Pyelonephritis, 74
salpingitis versus, 127
Pyogenic salpingitis, 124

Queyrat's erythroplasia, 113

Radiography, fetal maturity and, 79
Radiotherapy
cervical carcinoma and, 146
endometrial carcinoma and, 160
Rectourethral fistula, 3
Rectovesical fistula, 3
Reinke's albuminoid crystals, 171
Renal blood flow, 56
Renal disorder
amenorrhea and, 199–200
pyelonephritis and, 74
Renal ectopy, 2
Reproductive gynecology, 179–204
amenorrhea and, 184–191
dysfunctional uterine bleeding and, 194–202
dysmenorrhea and, 202–203
fertility and, 191–194
menopause and, 181–183
premenstrual tension syndrome and, 203–204
puberty and, 179–181
Resistant ovary syndrome, 187
Respiratory depression, 60

Respiratory distress syndrome, 93–94
diabetes and, 69
Respiratory system
lecithin/sphingomyelin ratio and, 78
neonatal assessment of, 38
pregnancy and, 14
Restitution, delivery and, 33
Resuscitation, neonatal, 37
Retained placenta, 51
Retardation, intrauterine growth, 84
$Rh^+$ antigen, 63
Rh blood group incompatibility, 61–64
Rh immunoglobulin, 42
Ritgen procedure, 33
Ritodrine, 92, 93
Rotation, delivery and, 33–34
Round ligament syndrome, 29
Rubella immunization, 42
Rupture
amniotic membranes and
labor and, 32
premature, 95–97
marginal sinus and, 46, 48

Salbutomol, 93
Salpingitis, 124–132
Sarcomatous fibroid, 151
Scalp blood, 76
Schiller test, 145
Schistosomiasis, 187–188
Screen-film mammography, 139
Screening for breast carcinoma, 139–141
Sebaceous cyst, 118
Seborrheic keratitis, 108
Secondary dysmenorrhea, 123–136

Secondary sex cord, 4
Secretion, nipple, 140
Seizure, 59–60
  eclaptic, 56
Semen analysis, 193
Septum
  cardiac, 72
  urorectal, 3
Serous borderline papillary
    cystadenocarcinoma, 165
Serous cystadenoma, 164
Sertoli-Leydig cell tumor, 171–172
Sertoli support cells, 4
Sex, chromosomal, 3
Sex cord, 4
Sexuality, 223–226
Sexually transmitted disease, 110, 112
SFH. *See* Symphysis-fundal height
SGA. *See* Small for gestational age
Sheath, visceral and muscle, 138
Sheehan's syndrome, 48
Sign
  Chadwick's, 20
  Goddell's, 22
  Hegar's, 22
  Piskacek's, 22
  Spalding's, 25
Single follicle cyst, 168–169
Sinus, marginal, 46, 48
Skin
  neonatal assessment of, 38
  oral contraceptive and, 210–211
  pregnancy and, 20
Small for gestational age (SGA), 90
Smear, Papanicolaou, 145
Sonography. *See* Ultrasound
Spalding's sign, 25

Spermatogenesis, 192
Spinnbarkeit, 196
Spontaneous rupture of amniotic mem-
    branes (SROM), 32
Squamous cell carcinoma
  cervical, 141
  vaginal, 123
SROM. *See* Spontaneous rupture of
    amniotic membranes
Stein-Leventhal syndrome, 155
  dysfunctional uterine bleeding and,
    198
Stenosis, valvular, 72
Sterilization, 215–218, 219
Steroid
  endometriosis and, 134
  oral contraceptive and, 211
  respiratory distress syndrome and,
    94
Stress, amenorrhea and, 190–191
Stress test of fetal well-being, 79–82
Striae, atrophic, 20
Stroma, ovarian neoplasm of, 176–
    177
Struma ovarii, 175
Submucosal myoma, 150
Suckling, 39–40
Suctioning, neonatal, 34–35
Sulfonamide, 74
Superfecundation, 99
Superfetation, 99
Surgically corrected heart disease, 73–
    74
Sweat gland adenitis, 111
Symphisis-fundal height (SFH), 22
Symphysis-fundal height (SFH)
  prenatal history and, 26

Tanner stages, 179
Tap, amniocentesis, 76–77
Telogen effluvium, 21
Teratoma, 176
Teratomatous germ cell tumor, 174–176
Term birth, 25
Testicular biopsy, 193
Testicular tissue, 7
Tetracycline
  fetus and, 74
  urethritis and, 113
Theca-lutein cyst, 169–170
Thecoma, 171
Thelarch, 179
Thiazide diuretic, 57
Thrombocytopenia, 57
Thyroid-stimulating hormone (TSH), 23
Tocolytic drug, 92, 93
Torsion, adnexal, 128
Traction of placenta, 50
Transfusion, exchange, 62–63
Trauma
  postpartum hemorrhage and, 50
  uterovaginal prolapse and, 137–139
*Treponema pallidum*, 116
*Trichomonas vaginalis*, 120
Triplets, 100
Trophoblastic disease, gestational, 100–105
TSH. *See* Thyroid-stimulating hormone
Tubal ligation, 215, 217
Tube, fallopian
  infertility and, 192–193
  inflammation of, 124–132

Tubercles, Montgomery's, 20
Tubercular infection, 187–188
Tubercular salpingitis, 131–132
Tubule, mesonephric, 7
Tumor. *See* Malignancy
Twins, 98

Ulcerative disorder, 107, 109
Ultrasound
  breast and, 141
  fetopelvic, 78
  pregnancy and, 83–84
    ectopic, 135–136
Umbilical cord
  delivery and, 33
  prolapse of, 89–90
*Ureaplasma ureolyticum*, 125
Ureter, 3
Ureteric bud, 1
Urethral disease, 113
Urethritis, 113
  menopause and, 183
Urethrocoele, 138
Urinary bladder irritability, 21
Urorectal septum, 3
Uterine bleeding, dysfunctional, 195–204
Uterine insufficiency, 85, 87
  hypotonic, 85
Uterovaginal prolapse, 137–139
Uterus
  atony and, 50
  fundus and, 41
  infertility and, 193
  postpartum period and, 38
  pregnancy and, 22

Vagina, 117–123
  mucosal discoloration of, 20
  oral contraceptive effects and, 209
  prenatal examination and, 27
Vaginal bleeding
  postmenopausal, 159
  pregnancy and, 43–53, 201–202
Vaginitis, 118–122
  pregnancy and, 21
Valvular disease, cardiac, 72
Varicosity, 20
Vasa previa, 46, 48
Vascular changes in pregnancy, 20
Vasectomy, 217–218, 219
Venous plasma glucose (VPG), 66
Venous varicosity, 20
Vesicourethral unit, 3
Vestibular gland adenitis, 111
Villus
  choriocarcinoma and, 102
  hydatidiform mole and, 101
Viral sexually transmitted disease, 112
Virilization, 7, 9–12
  Sertoli-Leydig cell tumor and, 172

Visceral sheath, 138
Visual disturbances, 57
Vital signs, neonatal, 38
VPG. *See* Venous plasma glucose
Vulva, 107–119
  neoplasia and, 118–119

Warfarin, 74
Weight
  hypertension and, 26
  menstruation and, 198
  neonatal, 90
  pregnancy and, 13
White lesions, vulvar, 109–110
Wolffian duct, 3

Xeroradiography, 139
X,Y mosaicism, 189

Yolk sac, 4

Clomiphene Citrate = acts by competing $\bar{c}$ endogenous circulating estrogens for estrogen binding sites in the hypothalamus, and ∴ blocking the $n\ell$ ⊘ Feedback of endog estrogens + permits release of GnRH

Danazol = a progestational compound derived from testosterone. It induces a pseudo-menopause, but does not alter basal GnRH levels. Appears to act as an antiestrogen + will cause endometrial atrophy. Cyclic menses return almost immed upon withdrawal.

OCP: Progesterone suppresses LH secretion while estrogen suppresses FSH secretion. The prog. effect will always take precedence over the estrogenic effect unless estrogen dose is ↑ alot.

Stranguary ≡ difficulty in micturition, the urine being passed drop by drop c̄ pain + tenesmus.

molimen≡ an effort; the laborious performance of a nl function

pessary ≡ medicated vaginal supp.

ectropion ≡ A rolling outward of the margin of a part

chloasma ≡ occurrence of extensive brown patches of irregular shape + size on the skin of face + elsewhere Assoc c̄ pregnancy, menopause, OCPs.

galactorrhea ≡ Nonpuerpal secretion from breast of watery or milky fluid that contains neither pus nor blood.

Triad of major complications of Pregnancy:
① Preg-induced HTN
② Sepsis
③ hemorrhage

lie - refers to the relation of the long axis of Fetus to that of the mother. Longitudinal, transverse or oblique.
Attitude - Fetal Posture - Flexed/extended
Presentation - Portion of Baby Foremost in birth canal

p113   strangury
p210   chloasma
p138   pessaries
p192   molimina
p200   ectropion

# Staging of Ovarian cA

**stage I**    Growth limited to ovary

   a) limited to 1 ovary; No ascites. No tumor on ext surface. capsule intact.

   b) limited to both ovaries: No ascites. No tumor on ext surface, capsule intact

   c) @ but c̄ tumor on surface of 1 or both ov. or c̄ capsule rupture; or c̄ ascites present containing malig cells or c̄ ⊕ peritoneal washing

**stage II**    Growth involving 1 or both ovaries c̄ pelvic extension.

   a) Extension +1or mets to uterus +1or tubes

   b) Extension to other pelvic tissues,

   c) @ but c̄ tumor on surf of 1 or both ov. or c̄ capsule rupture; or c̄ ascites present containing malignant cells or c̄ ⊕ peritoneal washings

**stage III**    Tumor involving 1 or both ovaries c̄ peritum implants outside the pelvis +1or ⊕ retroperitoneal or inguinal nodes. superficial liver mets,= stage III. Tumor is limited to the true pelvis but c̄ histo proved malignant extension to small bowel or omentum

   a) Grossly limited to true pelvis c̄ ∅ nodes, but c̄ histo confirmed micro seeding of abd peritoneal seeding.

   b) of 1 or both ovaries ō histo confirmed implants of Abd peritoneal surfaces, none exceeding 2 cm in diameter. ∅ nodes.

   c) Abd implants > 2cm +1or ⊕ retroperitoneal or inguinal nodes.

**stage IV**    1 or both ovaries c̄ distant mets. If pleural effussions present, must get ⊕ cytology Parenchymal liver mets = IV.

# Endometrial CA surgical staging

**Distribution**

stage I : Depth of Invasion : Corpus

75% 
  A. Endometrium
  B. Inner ½ myometrium
  C. Outer ½ "

stage II : DoI : endo cervix

9-10%
  A. epithelium of Cx
  B. stroma of Cx

stage III :

5%
  A. Adnexal ⊕ Peritoneal cytology
  B. vaginal mets
  C. Pelvic / para-aortic nodes

stage IV

5%
  A. Bladder / Rectal mucosa
  B. Distant mets

---

| | Complete Mole | Partial Mole |
|---|---|---|
| | 46, XX | Triploid |
| Edema: | All villi | Some villi |
| Tropho. Prolif | Diffuse; circumf. | Focal: slight |
| | Atypia often present | Absent |
| serum hCG elevated | | Less |
| Tissue hCG 3+ | | 1+ |
| | 2% → Chorio Ca | rare → Chorio Ca |

CA of Cervix

FSH → granulosa cell proliferation & estrogen
synthesis, acc of antral fluid + induction
of LH receptors. All leading to graafian
follicle formation which secretes large
amts of estrogen into circulation, which
triggers release of LH → ruputure of follicle,
expulsion of egg + formation of corpus
luteum.

PSF
Danforth
on g cells →

Theca cells are LH responsive. Theca-lutein cysts
are often assoc c̄ molar preg since the
excessive βHCG has LH activity. T-L cysts are
often bilateral.

---

Cervical CA staging
stage O:    CIS
Stage I:    Confined to Cx
    Ia.  microinvasion
        Ia₁. <1mm stromal invasion
        Ia₂. 1-5mm deep. No >7mm wide
    Ib  greater than Ia₂. >5mm still in Cx.
        Ib₁. occult. Not clinically visible
        Ib₂ All others limited to uterus
stage II:  Ca extends beyond Cx Not to Pelvic
           side wall.
    IIa  Involves upper 2/3 of vagina. No
         obvious parametrial involvement
    IIb  Parametrial involvement not to side wall
stage III: Ca extends onto pelvic side wall or lower
           1/3 of vagina or any ureter involvement.
    IIIa: Lower 1/3 vagina. Not to PSW.
    IIIb: To pelvic side wall
stage IV   mucosa of bladder/rectum
    IVa: adj organs
    IVb: distant organs.